Dirk Schweigler

Histamine intolerance

from a totally new perspective

The author has carefully selected and reviewed the advice provided in this book. However, it should in no way replace getting competent medical advice. All information in this book is therefore provided without any warranty or guarantee of any kind on the part of the author. The author's liability for personal injury, property damage and financial loss is also excluded.

First edition 2025
Copyright © 2025 Dirk Schweigler

Illustrations: *Shutterstock*
Translation: *Mary Burdman, PA, USA*

Table of contents

Introduction

Almost everyone of us has had a painful experience with histamine already: A brief touch of a stinging nettle is already enough. These otherwise harmony-seeking little plants inject histamine on contact into the skin with their fine hairs and the subsequent reaction is pretty obvious: The skin reacts to this with itching and a rash.

However, histamine is more than just a component of nettles. It fulfills many important tasks in our body, but if certain things are out of balance, histamine can quickly become a problem.

Especially in the beginning, most people don´t even know where their strange symptoms such as a rash, runny nose or digestive problems are coming from. Therefore, the most important step is to find out if histamine intolerance is the reason behind these symptoms. In the following, we will take a closer look at how to determine histamine intolerance.

If you already know for sure that histamine intolerance is the reason for your digestive problems, then you naturally want to get rid of this intolerance as quickly as possible. Unfortunately, conventional medicine does not provide a sufficient answer to the question "How can I get rid of my histamine intolerance?" You usually only get the advice that you should avoid histamine-rich foods and live with it, possibly for the rest of your life.

In the title, I have announced a completely new perspective on histamine intolerance and you have probably been wondering what this is about. I myself had to struggle with digestive and severe histamine problems for a long time. To get rid of my complaints, I have read many books on this subject and have done intensive research.

While I was getting deeper and deeper into the topic of histamine intolerance, I have noticed that the vast majority of information only deals with how to avoid histamine-rich foods or how to live with the disease. The result is always the same: You have to endure histamine intolerance for the rest of your life.

That is why I would like to bring a completely new perspective on the subject of histamine intolerance into play – it is the perspective of the **causes**. You shouldn't have to be concerned with how to come to terms with your symptoms for the rest of your life. Instead, the goal is to get rid of them. The general principle behind this is very simple: If you cure the cause of a disease, the symptoms will disappear all by themselves. However, this principle won't work the other way around.

One day, I was watching the movie "Vantage Point" and I was fascinated with the way it tells one story from many different perspectives. In the movie, the heads of state of several countries meet for an anti-terrorist summit. At this meeting, there is an assassination attempt against the U.S. president and the movie continues telling the story from eight different perspectives: From the view of a woman reporter, a police officer, a spectator, from the perspective of the U.S. president and from the instigators of the terrorist act.

I find this approach very interesting, because a story is not the only thing we can see from several vantage points, but a disease also has several perspectives. Therefore, I would not only like to look at the symptoms of histamine intolerance, but I would rather bring the focus to the causes. The causes are considered far too rarely, even though they are the root of the problem.

The subject of histamine is not so simple in itself. This is because there are various reasons why histamine intolerance can develop. One person may have a copper or vitamin B6 deficiency, the next may have histamine problems due to a damaged intestine and a third may have been exposed to heavy metals.

That is why there won't ever be a single pill that suddenly makes all the symptoms disappear. There are simply far too many possible causes and if it were so easy to cure histamine intolerance, there wouldn't be so many people still suffering from it. Highly complex processes take place in our body every day and that is why there are so many different reasons for developing histamine intolerance.

Even if the whole topic is not that simple and seems confusing in the beginning, I would like to encourage you at this point, because there are many possible therapies for histamine intolerance and there is a lot that you can do about it. These therapies, which I will introduce later, directly address to the cause of the problem.

There is a very fundamental rule that applies to all diseases and histamine intolerance in particular: First the diagnosis, then the treatment! You don't start with just taking a pill and hope that it might help somehow. That would be a bit like going on vacation by car without having a map.

Instead, the correct approach is to first measure certain values via a blood, stool or urine sample. This shows you exactly where something is out of kilter in your body. Only then comes the treatment, which will start precisely by dealing with this very specific problem.

Fortunately, you are not completely on your own in the search for the cause, because modern laboratory medicine nowadays opens up undreamt-of possibilities. You just have to be aware of these possibilities and use them. *Chapter 3* will take a closer look at which tests are very useful to detect the causes.

My own search for a solution was a very long road and I often experienced setbacks. However, after many tests and therapies, I have overcome my digestive problems and I can eat almost everything again now. During that time, I have tried and tested almost all the measures recommended in this book myself.

Since I have been working for many years as a scientist in a hospital, it is very important to me that any test or treatment is always scientific. In the 21st century, the scientific methods available are simply far too good. These work excellently, so there is no need to use dubious, unverifiable methods.

However, in addition to science, the experiences of other people with histamine intolerance are very important as well. The topic of histamine intolerance is still quite new and there are hardly any research results on it – at least as far as healing is concerned. That is why we shouldn´t just to grey theory. The actual experiences of others are very important and therefore I have tried to include a lot of them here.

1 What exactly is this mysterious histamine?

Histamine is always produced when proteins are broken down or transformed [1]. It doesn´t occur only in foods or beverages, but a lot is produced within our body. The body can store histamine in cells and it is used to fulfill specific functions. Once the body´s own histamine has fulfilled its purpose, this histamine is broken down and excreted.

As we can see, histamine is not generally a bad thing at all. It only becomes problematic when excessive histamine is produced in the body or when it can´t be properly broken down. In both cases, we are then speaking of histamine intolerance. That means everybody has histamine in their body and additionally consumes it with food. This is totally normal. It only becomes a problem when there is too much of histamine in the body that can´t be broken down.

A brief look at the statistics shows that about 80% of those who suffer from histamine intolerance are women, and most of them are 40 years or older. One reason could be the hormonal changes in women at a certain age. Another reason why more women than men suffer from histamine intolerance may be that they are more health conscious. Their unclear digestive problems are then diagnosed as histamine intolerance.

One important factor is the breakdown of histamine in the body, but this does not only depend on one single factor. There are multiple reasons for impaired breakdown of histamine, such as the condition of the intestine, the balance of hormones or a deficiency of certain nutrients.

As already described, histamine is not only a nuisance, but it also has **very important tasks** to perform in the body. These include

✓ Stimulation of gastric acid production
✓ Regulation of the sleep-wake rhythm
✓ Increase the movement of the intestine
✓ Regulation of body temperature
✓ Defense against exogenous substances
✓ Regulation of blood pressure

From a biological point of view, histamine belongs to the group of **biogenic amines**. They are formed during the conversion of amino acids. Besides histamine, there are other biogenic amines such as cadaverine, serotonin and tyramine. During the degradation process, a kind of competition sometimes arises, because one enzyme is needed for degrading multiple biogenic amines.

The histamine in our body is mainly broken down by the DAO enzyme. If a meal contains not only histamine but various biogenic amines, the DAO enzyme has its hands full. In addition to histamine, it must also take care of the breakdown of other biogenic amines.

If the DAO enzyme is busy breaking down another biogenic amine, there is not much left to break down histamine. The histamine must therefore take a back seat. For this reason, a food can be unfavorable for histamine sufferers, even though it actually contains very little or no histamine. The reason behind this is that other biogenic amines in this food are broken down even before the histamine and thus there is too little of the DAO enzyme left to break down the histamine.

The topic of biogenic amines makes the issue of histamine even more complicated. However, in order not to make things too complicated, it is only crucial that you don't just look at the histamine content of a food alone. The most important thing is that you listen to your body about whether you can digest a food well or not.

1.1   The delicate histamine balance

Every day, we come into contact with histamine several times, because histamine is found in many foods and the body also produces it. As mentioned before, histamine in itself is nothing bad or harmful for us. Only too much of it can lead to problems.

If histamine is produced by the body itself, it is called endogenous histamine. However, there is not just one place in the body where histamine arises – it can be produced almost anywhere. Depending on the organ, this task is done by different cells, such as ECL cells or mast cells. This means, that the body can produce histamine in the stomach, in the intestine or in the brain and it can also store it there.

This is the reason why the symptoms can be so different for each person. Histamine can occur anywhere in the body and while one person complains of headaches or redness in the face, it affects the digestion of another.

In a healthy person, the body only releases histamine when it is really needed – for example, to regulate blood pressure or to initiate an inflammation at a particular site. However, this process can get out of hand when the stored histamine is released in an uncontrolled way, for example by certain drugs.

In addition to the histamine stored in the body, additional amounts of histamine enter the body through our food. This is normal and does not cause any problems in a healthy person, because the histamine is broken down by certain enzymes.

There is not an infinite number of enzymes that are responsible for the degradation of histamine: **HNMT** (Histamine N-Methyltransferase), which degrades histamine inside the cells and the second one is **DAO** (diamine oxidase) which degrades histamine outside the cells. Both enzymes are active throughout our body, but DAO takes over most of the histamine breakdown process.

The DAO enzyme is mainly produced in the cells of the intestine [2]. This also explains why an impaired intestine often occurs together with histamine intolerance. If the intestine is not doing well, then too little DAO is produced and histamine cannot be broken down properly due to the lack of DAO.

In the body, there is a perpetual up and down between the ingestion or production of histamine on the one side and the subsequent breakdown of histamine on the other side. However, breaking down histamine does not work smoothly for everyone, because it involves a complex interaction of many factors.

Unfortunately, there is no maximum level of histamine at which every person has problems. For example, you can't say that all people with a histamine intolerance have problems exactly after consuming 50 grams of cheese. Instead, everyone has an **individual tolerance limit** that determines how much histamine you can tolerate. This tolerance limit can change over time, since it depends on hormones, the intestinal flora or stress.

But it is not just about the amount, tolerance of the exact same food can also differ for everyone. While one person might be fine with a glass of red wine, someone else gets a severe headache from it, because there is just too much histamine in it. There are certain guidelines about which foods and beverages might cause histamine problems. But in the end, everyone is individual and might react in a different way.

1.2   Symptoms: How do you notice histamine?

When you have a cold, you normally get the typical symptoms such as feeling listless, feverish or coughing. A histamine disease, on the other hand, is not so easy to recognize. This is because there are many receptors in the body where histamine can dock on. Accordingly, due to the variety of different places and receptors, symptoms can also occur in very different places.

However, there are some typical histamine symptoms that recur frequently:

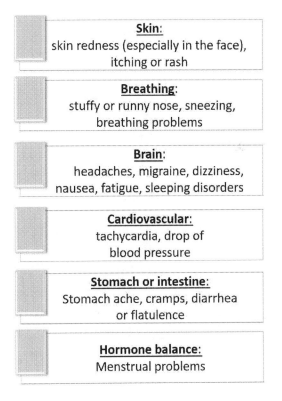

Skin:
skin redness (especially in the face),
itching or rash

Breathing:
stuffy or runny nose, sneezing,
breathing problems

Brain:
headaches, migraine, dizziness,
nausea, fatigue, sleeping disorders

Cardiovascular:
tachycardia, drop of
blood pressure

Stomach or intestine:
Stomach ache, cramps, diarrhea
or flatulence

Hormone balance:
Menstrual problems

It is no coincidence that precisely these symptoms occur due to histamine intolerance. Let´s take a closer look at why the skin reddens after a histamine-rich meal. When too much histamine is circulating in the body, the blood vessels are dilated. This allows more blood to flow through the vessels and the affected skin areas are supplied with more blood. This in turn leads to reddening of the skin from histamine.

Furthermore, abdominal pain and diarrhea are also typical symptoms of histamine intolerance. Histamine stimulates the smooth muscles in the body. Smooth muscle fibers are generally found in parts of the body we cannot influence consciously, for example the heartbeat or digestion in the gastrointestinal tract [3]. When these muscles are stimulated by histamine, they can get tense (abdominal cramps) or they start to transport food very quickly (diarrhea).

The time after a meal when histamine begins to become active can also be very different for each person. Histamine release can occur already in the stomach. If the stomach reacts to the histamine overdose, then these symptoms are usually noticeable just a few minutes after the meal.

However, it is also possible that the histamine causes problems later in the intestine. The noticeable symptoms take much longer, because the food needs a certain amount of time before it even reaches the intestine. Liquids and light food are digested quickly by the stomach, whereas certain foods such as meat take much longer. It can happen that a meal lies in the stomach for more than five hours and only then gradually travels into the intestine.

When histamine causes problems in the intestine, the symptoms appear within a significant time lag after eating, sometimes even on the next day. This makes it particularly difficult to find out which food is causing you trouble. When digestive problems show up after breakfast, then you might not think that this could actually be from your evening meal, but that's possible. The time gap between eating and experiencing the symptoms can range from a few minutes to more than 24 hours.

When you want to find out if you are suffering from histamine intolerance, one option is to use laboratory values. These lab values are reliable, but they are not always the whole truth. However, there is a way that will produce a very clear result when you want to test if you have histamine intolerance: It is the **elimination diet**. This kind of diet requires avoiding histamine-rich foods for about two to three weeks. If you feel much better during this time or if the symptoms even disappear completely, then it is very likely that you have histamine intolerance.

Nevertheless, it is not only food that can create a histamine surplus in the body. **Allergies** such as house dust or animal hair allergies can also lead to massive release of histamine. When the body comes into contact with substances to which it is allergic to, it releases histamine. This reaction is regardless of whether the histamine release was due to an allergic reaction to food, pollen or animal hair.

The topic of allergy and histamine release is a good illustration of how everything in the body is closely interrelated. The immune system is very important in the development of allergies. If the immune system suddenly classifies harmless substances such as pollen or animal hair as hostile, an allergic reaction begins. This allergic reaction in turn releases new histamine.

Since more than 80% of the immune system is located in the intestine, a large number of immune defense cells are produced here. This means: When the intestine is in bad shape, the immune system suffers as well.

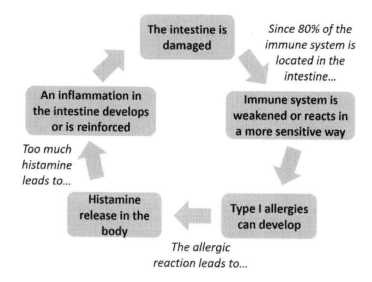

The histamine released by an allergy can affect the intestine and cause an inflammation in the intestine. From here on, the cycle starts all over again and it can even intensify. The worsened condition of the intestine affects the immune system and thus increases the possibility of more allergies.

1.3   The causes: What leads to histamine intolerance?

Most people wonder *"Where did I actually get my histamine intolerance from"*? This question is always very exciting, but in most cases, it is no longer possible to say what the exact trigger was. You don't go to bed totally healthy and next day wake up with a completely damaged intestine or histamine intolerance. Such an illness usually creeps up on you slowly. Over weeks and months, it gets worse and worse, bit by bit, without there having been a noticeable "boom" event beforehand.

As already mentioned, to get rid of the histamine disease, you always have to look for the root cause. Let's assume you had a severe intestinal infection in the past. Since then, you have noticed histamine symptoms and you have a feeling that your intestine is completely out of balance. If the initial infection has completely disappeared in the meantime, then you "only" have to take care of building up your intestinal flora in order to become healthy again.

In this example, it would be great to know which virus was the trigger and where you got it from. However, that is not really important anymore, since the virus is gone and that means that the cause of the disease is gone as well. You only have to clean up and get your intestine back in balance again.

But what if the actual trigger has not disappeared yet and it is still sitting in your body. Then you have to find this trigger and eliminate it, because as long as the problem is still dormant in your body, the symptoms will not go away. It is the age-old principle of cause and symptom.

But what exactly is meant by symptoms? Symptoms are all sensations that we can see or feel: An itch on the skin, a runny nose, headache, fatigue or abdominal pain. You don't really need a doctor to identify your symptoms, because you deal with them every day. Identifying the symptoms is the easiest part, but after that the really crucial questions arise: What is going wrong in my body so that my health is suddenly on a roller coaster? And what is the root cause of these symptoms?

These questions are the start of the path on which the search for the causes begins. If you can eliminate the cause, then the annoying symptoms will automatically go away. It doesn't work the other way around: You can work on your symptoms for the rest of your life, but the disease won't go away. For example, using a hot water bottle to ease abdominal cramps may be pleasant, but in the end, it does not help against the cause. It only alleviates the symptoms for a while.

The basic principle of cause and symptoms says that something in your body is out of balance (this is the cause) and that cause is the reason why you are having certain symptoms. In order to get rid of these disorders, we need to take a closer look at the causes. In contrast to the symptoms, you can neither see nor feel the causes. But with today's state-of-the-art laboratory medicine, you can check for them and this is an invaluable advantage.

Now, it would be so wonderfully simple if I could tell you that there is only one single cause of histamine disease. However, if it were that simple, then your doctor or gastroenterologist would have already helped and you would not have to worry about it yourself.

However, the number of possible causes for histamine intolerance is manageable:

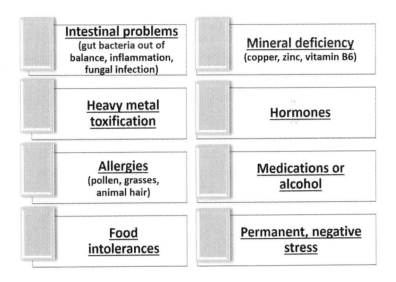

In order to make a good progress in healing and in finding the cause of your histamine intolerance, you can´t get around measuring certain lab values. When you are new to the topic of histamine intolerance, these lab terms can scare you off really quickly. I wonder if some scientists sit in their labs and joke around: "Let's see if we can confuse people with terms like *alpha-1 antitrypsin* or *secretory immunoglobulin A*?"

However, we have to get through this, because it is very important to understand what is behind these terms. Only then will you be able to get to the root cause of your histamine disease. In *Chapter 3*, we will then take a closer look at each single cause and how to treat it.

We have gone a little deeper now into the difference between cause and symptom and I would like to emphasize again: The most important thing, when it comes to healing any disease, is to understand the difference between the symptom and the underlying cause. Strangely enough, even doctors hardly seem to know the difference between symptom and cause when it comes to histamine intolerance. In many cases, only an antihistamine is prescribed against the symptoms and only very few doctors will investigate to find the root cause.

During the years of searching for a solution for my histamine problems, I met many people with digestive disorders for whom their doctor was unable to provide any help at all. Additionally, the health insurance companies are totally unconcerned as well.

I would like to give you a little example from Germany: With the exception of a colonoscopy or a standard blood count, almost none of the costs for an examination for histamine intolerance are covered by the statutory health insurance. Unfortunately, this leaves patients to fend for themselves. Health insurers in particular should be very interested in seeing that insured patients take care of their health. Above all, they should support those who really want to actively do something for their health.

I can think of at least 10 scientific tests which are extremely helpful for finding the cause of histamine intolerance and digestive disorders. These tests are conducted by accredited laboratories, where doctors also send their samples, yet these tests for histamine are still not covered and accepted by health insurance. For most people, especially those with lower incomes, it would make a fundamental difference to become healthy if insurance companies would support them financially.

However, you shouldn't get too annoyed about this issue, because otherwise your pulse and histamine level will only rise unnecessarily. Fortunately, you don't have to rely on the statutory health insurance companies alone; there are some good ways to get some support for these examinations. More about this in Chapter *4.3 Making your piggy bank happy: Financial tips & ideas.*

2 Nutrition – What can I still eat despite my histamine intolerance?

A good treatment is very important to get back on track healthwise. Nevertheless, there is something else that contributes at least as much to healing as a good treatment does and that is **everyday lifestyle as well as diet**.

You can swallow the most fantastic pills – they will hardly help, if you take too little care of your health in everyday life. Of course, there are temptations to give in and eat sweets or delicious food, even if it is rich in histamine. A good meal is more than just nutritional intake; it also touches the soul and it is not all that dramatic to give in to a craving for chocolate or a glass of alcohol every once in a while. It is more the **sum of all sins** which is decisive. Especially in case of histamine intolerance and digestive problems, you should be much stricter in your daily lifestyle and your diet than a healthy person has to be. That´s the reason why it is so important to constantly keep an eye on your daily habits and improve them, step by step.

Nutrition in particular is very important in this context and this does not just mean avoiding histamine. Even for a healthy person, nutrition is very important, because it builds up all cells of which we are made. Unfortunately, the topic of nutrition is anything but simple in the case of histamine intolerance. There are so many pitfalls and exceptions that sometimes you hardly know what you are allowed to eat and what not.

In the following, we will therefore look at which foods can be tolerated if you have histamine intolerance and which should be avoided. Furthermore, you will learn some nutritional basics, which are generally helpful for digestive problems.

2.1   Food under the histamine magnifying glass

For people with histamine intolerance, diet is really the key! If you keep eating foods you can't tolerate, then your gut and your whole digestive system will not get any rest and will keep getting irritated over and over again.

When the intestine can´t calm down, inflammations cannot heal, the intestinal flora does not regain its balance and the pH value in the intestine shifts. You have to give your body the chance to recover – and that can only be done with a low-histamine diet for the time being.

In the real estate industry, there are three factors that are particularly important when buying a house. These factors have long been known among real estate agents and they are in descending order: location, location and location. This hints a bit that the location of a house is a very important factor when buying real estate.

For histamine intolerance, there are also three important rules that you should follow. These rules are in descending order: freshness, freshness and again ... you guess it ... freshness! The length of time a food has been stored is extremely important for the creation of histamine. The fresher a food, the lower its histamine content usually is.

To make this clearer, let us take a closer look at fish. Shortly after being caught, fish contains almost no histamine at all. It is therefore well tolerated. However, after just a few hours, enormous amounts of histamine will have formed if the fish is not frozen immediately. The fish is then far from having gone bad. It is still edible and won´t cause any problems for healthy people. Just the histamine level has increased and might cause problems for people with histamine intolerance.

The example of fish shows very well that we cannot make any general statements at all about the histamine content in food. The amount of histamine can fluctuate enormously within a short period of time and this is exactly the reason why diet and selecting the right food is so difficult at the beginning.

With lactose intolerance, the issue of nutrition is much easier. The lactose content in a food remains constant, regardless of whether you eat it immediately after it is produced or a few days later. It is similar with fructose intolerance or gluten intolerance.

Nevertheless, with a little experience, you will be able to recognize histamine-containing foods very well. Nowadays, there are many digital helpers that allow you to get good information about the histamine level of certain foods – even when you're on the road.

The decisive factor is to know in the first place that you are not suffering from some inexplicable intestinal problem, but that histamine intolerance is behind your symptoms. Once you have figured this out, then you have to find the cause of your histamine intolerance in order to feel better and get rid of the symptoms.

For buying and also for preparing food, there are a few basic rules regarding histamine:

√ Don't buy food that is close to the expiration date

√ Don't store leftover food too long and eat it as soon as possible

√ Deep-frozen food has advantages, when the deep-freezing chain wasn't interrupted

√ Buy food fresh and multiple times per week instead of bulk shopping

Even if the food markets offer great price bargains when the food is about to expire, this is not a good thing for someone with histamine intolerance. The price is only discounted because the food is already somewhat older and will expire soon.

If the "best-before" date of a food is about to expire, then this food is no longer very fresh and may accordingly already contain a lot of histamine. For people without histamine intolerance, this is not a problem at all and it is a good thing not to throw food away. However, if you have histamine intolerance you should select food that is as fresh as possible.

This is especially true for meat, fish, cheese and many other goods from the refrigerated shelf.

If you have cooked a large amount at home and save the rest, then the leftovers should be eaten as soon as possible. It would not be good to eat it even just after three or four days. Meanwhile, the histamine content has increased significantly. The sooner you eat the leftover portion, the less histamine can emerge. At this point, I would like to point out once again that there are no fixed specifications for storage time and the resulting histamine amounts. How long something can be stored and still be tolerated is completely different for every food and every person.

There are simply too many factors that come together: Each food develops histamine at a very different rate and every person has their very own tolerance limit. This tolerance limit also fluctuates every day, depending on hormones, stress, the current state of the intestine and other foods that you have eaten.

That is why there is no information on how long you can store food in general in terms of histamine. You simply have to test out for yourself, which limits work well for you. However, the basic rule always applies: The histamine content increases the longer you store a food. In other words: The fresher, the better!

If you have cooked a little too much and you don´t want to eat the same thing again for the next couple days, then freezing is the better option than storing it in the refrigerator. Freezing does not eliminate the histamine that is already present in the food. However, due to the extremely low temperatures, the histamine-forming bacteria become inactive and they form significantly less histamine during the time in the freezer. When you want to eat the frozen food later, then thawing time should be kept very brief or avoided altogether, because the histamine-forming bacteria become active again very quickly during thawing and continue their work tirelessly.

Frozen food generally has one major disadvantage compared to fresh food: Freezing reduces the number of enzymes. The same happens on the other side of the temperature scale as well, when you are heating food. This also destroys the enzymes. They are a very important component, especially in fruits and vegetables and they are almost as important as vitamins and minerals.

Therefore, unprocessed and short-stored foods are ideal. However, even if freezing destroys enzymes in the food, it can help to slow down the process of histamine formation and that is very important for everyone who has histamine intolerance.

As mentioned before, freshness is very crucial when it comes to histamine and that's why you should avoid bulk shopping, at least as far as certain foods are concerned. Of course, you can still buy paper towels or toothbrushes many weeks in advance. However, for certain foods, it is better that you go shopping two to three times a week to buy them as fresh as possible.

For example, if you buy meat on Monday but you don't prepare it until Thursday, then there are three days in between when bacteria can produce a lot of histamine from the amino acid *"histidine."*

Therefore, certain foods should be purchased on the same day of preparation, or at most one day before. Of course, it's annoying to shop more often than you're actually used to, but it is of no use to only go shopping once a week while the rest of the week you are constantly struggling with histamine and digestive problems.

In terms of its structure, histamine is a bit like a superhero: It is indestructible. You can boil it at over 100°C for hours – it will survive. You can also freeze it at -18°C in your freezer – that doesn't help either. You cannot extract the amount of histamine once it's in a food. In short, histamine is so stable that it **cannot be destroyed by either heating or freezing**.

Mostly, histamine is formed in protein-rich foods. This includes above all **meat and fish**. Histamine forms here over the duration of storage and the fresher you buy food, the less histamine it contains. However, large amounts of histamine are also found in fermented foods. These include long-aged cheese, pickled vegetables, wine or beer. Here, the histamine has already been formed by bacteria in the manufacturing process and these foods or beverages already arrive in the store with a lot of histamine. In this case, the time of storage does not make much of a difference since a large proportion of histamine is already in the food right after it is produced.

On the other hand, fats and oils are usually very well tolerated. In order to do something good for your health and to provide your body with many valuable nutrients, you should only consume high-quality fats, which support you with their good fatty acids.

High-quality fats are, for instance, **ghee, coconut oil and olive oil**. Inferior fats such as margarine, cheap rapeseed or sunflower oil should be avoided. For fats and oils, the time of storage is very important and they should not be stored for too long, since they are sensitive to light as well as oxygen. Therefore, it is advisable to buy smaller quantities of fats and oils rather than using a large bottle for several months or even years.

For alcoholic beverages, you simply have to try out your individual tolerance. More details on how alcohol and drugs can influence histamine intolerance will be found in *Chapter 3.7 Medications and alcohol.*

Now, you have probably been wondering all this time what exactly you can still eat despite your histamine intolerance. In the following, you will find some foods with an indication of whether they can be tolerated with histamine intolerance or not.

Of course, the overview does not include nearly all foods, but it is more intended to provide an initial overview. Smartphone apps are particularly helpful for making a detailed search right when you are shopping, at a restaurant or while cooking. There are databases that contain thousands of foods, and with an app on your phone, you have the information right when you need it.

Fish	
⊗	- Canned fish - Fish or seafood that is marinated, salted, dried, smoked or pickled in vinegar - Certain fish species like tuna, mackerel, herring, sardines or anchovies - Shellfish (mussel, crab, shrimp)
?	- *Fresh fish from supermarket* - *Seafood like mussels, squid, shrimp or crab*
✓	- Fresh fish from fish market - Frozen fish (defrost quickly) - Certain types of fish such as pollock, cod, trout or organic pangasius

	Meat and eggs
(✗)	- Canned meat - Cured, dried, marinated, smoked and generally preserved meat - Dried meat, raw ham, bacon and meat that has been hung for a long time - Almost all sausages: salami, liver sausage, bratwurst... - Finely chopped meat like spreads or meat
(?)	*- Very fresh meat*
(✓)	- Fresh meat of poultry, sheep, goat, beef, pork, wild boar, chicken thighs or turkey breast - Frozen meat (quick defrosting) - Eggs

	Dairy products and cheese
(✗)	- Emmental, Tilsit, Edam, ripe Camembert, Parmesan, mold-ripened cheese, raw milk cheese, cheese fondue or old Gouda
(?)	*- Raw milk, yogurt* *- Sour milk products: buttermilk, sour cream or feta cheese*
(✓)	- Pasteurized milk, long-life milk (UHT milk) - Butter, cream, whey - Fresh cheese: mozzarella, curd, cottage cheese, mascarpone, ricotta, fresh goat cheese - Young Gouda, butter cheese, unripened Camembert cheese

	Vegetable
⊗	- Spinach, tomatoes, ketchup or tomato juice, eggplants, avocados, olives - Legumes such as lentils and beans - Soy and soy products such as tofu - Pickled vegetables - Mushrooms: porcini, champignon
?	- *Olives without lactic fermentation* - *All mushrooms (except those mentioned above)*
✓	- All vegetables except those mentioned above

	Fruits
⊗	- Strawberries, raspberries, oranges or citrus fruits in general, bananas, pineapple, kiwis, pears, papayas, guavas
✓	- Apples, peaches, apricots, melons, mangos, cherries, sour cherries, blackberries, blueberries, cranberries, currants

	Cereals and bakery products
⊗	- Very fresh, warm baked goods
⦾?	- *Malt, wheat germ* - *Buckwheat*
✓	- Potatoes, corn, rice - Any processed forms: flour, baked goods or sauces - Crispbread, brown bread or you can make your own bread without yeast

	Oil, fats, nuts and seeds
⊗	- Nuts: Almost all types of nuts, especially walnuts, cashews, peanuts
✓	- All animal fats like butter or ghee - Almost all vegetable fats such as canola oil, olive oil, linseed oil, sunflower oil, coconut oil - Nuts: macadamia nuts, sweet chestnuts, coconut milk and coconut water

	Spices
⊗	- Almost all types of vinegar, especially wine vinegar and balsamic vinegar - Yeast extract, flavor enhancers (glutamate, sodium glutamate) - Bouillon, broth, soy sauce - Hot spices
✓	- Salt, garlic - Kitchen herbs (fresh and dried) and mild spices - Apple cider vinegar - Binding agents such as corn starch or potato starch

	Beverages
⊗	- Most alcoholic beverages - Soy milk - Energy drinks - Juices and soft drinks with incompatible
?	- *Rice milk, oat milk* - *Alcohol: clear spirits, non-alcoholic beer, wine or sparkling wine without histamine (can be ordered on the Internet)* - *Espresso, black tea, green tea, coffee*
✓	- Water - Herbal teas - Juices, fruit nectars and lemonades made from compatible ingredients - Almond milk

Sweets	
⊗	- Cocoa - Chocolate (milk chocolate and dark) - Nougat and marzipan
?	- *White chocolate*
✓	- Sugar, agave syrup, honey, stevia - Rice wafers

However, this table should only be used as a rough guide. If you can actually tolerate the main ingredient in a food, but it contains other ingredients as well, then suddenly you might not be able to tolerate the whole meal. For example, a portion of rice is usually fine with histamine intolerance. But if you have a sauce that comes with the rice and this sauce contains a lot of histamine, then you can get digestive problems. That's why you have to be very careful when you select your meals.

The same counts for fish or meat, if they are not as fresh as they appear when you buy them. All these tables about foods that are compatible with histamine intolerance are only pure theory. They can give a good hint, but in the end, your body decides if it can digest something well or not. Compared with other intolerances, it is not always easy to choose the right foods when you are histamine intolerant. Choosing tolerable food is more complex than if you are lactose or gluten intolerant.

Of course, you do not need to memorize the entire list. After a certain time, you will know the foods that you eat most often. At first, you might feel like you can't keep track of the incompatible foods at all. However, since you don't just eat one meal per week but obviously many more, you will quickly develop a routine for recognizing foods that are compatible and incompatible with histamine intolerance.

2.2   Tips for good nutrition

There are certain principles of nutrition that have been proven over many centuries. Most of them are well known, but surprisingly they are often forgotten.

A good balance is very important here: On the one hand, you should not restrict yourself too much in everyday life and banish all fun from life. A grumpy face every morning will not help in dealing with histamine intolerance at all. On the other hand, a certain amount of discipline is important for good health. With most things in life and especially with histamine intolerance, it is crucial to find the happy medium between discipline and enjoyment.

What you always have to keep in mind is that our bodies and the entirety human genetics did not just fall from the sky yesterday. Already hundreds of thousands of years ago, primates or Stone Age man had to assert themselves on a daily basis – against hunger, cold, bacteria, viruses and dangerous animals. Only those were able to adapt perfectly to these changing environmental conditions survived and reproduced. They then passed on these strong survival genes to their descendants.

If these genes proved successful in the children as well, then they also survived and were able to pass these good genes on to their children. On the other hand, the species that could not cope with the harsh environmental conditions eventually died out. We are therefore the result of extremely strict selection and carry the best survival genes within us.

It helps to know how the body has developed over thousands of years and that there is still a lot of Stone Age man in us. Just one or two generations of affluent living do not change the basic functions in our body.

However, what exactly does this whole historical development of humankind have to do with histamine disease? In order to become healthy again, it is not enough to simply avoid histamine. Rather, your entire lifestyle must be adapted and improved. This includes not only which foods you eat, but also what you deliberately don't eat, how much you sleep, how much you drink, if you smoke, how often you use medications and how often you exercise. All this and much more adds up to your overall health. Histamine is only one small part of the whole human work of art.

It seems there has been a trend over recent years that lifestyle gurus or fitness influencers want to tell us every day about the latest health trend or the food industry comes up with a new "superfood." In the end, you quickly lose track of all these trends and you will become confused about how to live a healthy life.

For anyone with histamine problems, it is best to forget such tips right away. These tips are only aimed at healthy people. For people with histamine intolerance, such claims can literally backfire. These self-proclaimed nutrition gurus are often only following the latest trends, which are set by huge companies. The food industry discovers a so-called "superfood" once again and it is praised to the skies. A short time later, the next superfood arrives on the scene.

However, there are certain dietary guidelines that have proven their worth over thousands of years. They can be found in the ancient books of traditional Chinese medicine (TCM) as well as in the scriptures of Ayurveda. The basics rules are consistent and completely independent of any trends or hypes.

The dietary rules of TCM and Ayurveda include which quantities of food you should eat at what time of the day, which foods are easily digestible, what are good and bad fatty acids and what effect proper chewing has on good digestion. Most of these guidelines apply to all people, whether you have a food intolerance or not.

The saying "*You are what you eat*" has been true for a long time. Everything that goes into our mouth is processed into what we are: Brain and nerve cells, skin, bones, blood, teeth and so on. Simply everything that creates us, physically and mentally, we gain to a large extent from food.

However, there are now several million people with food intolerances out there, and that is why the saying should nowadays be changed into *"You are what you can digest well."*

Very important are the small and simple things that the body needs: Lots of movement, fresh air, a balanced diet, harmonious relationships, and so on. Especially with histamine and intestinal problems, a healthy lifestyle is extremely important in order to recover. That is why we'll take a closer look at the most important lifestyle factors.

There is an old proverb when it comes to eating: "In the morning like an emperor, at noon like a king, and in the evening like a beggar". This describes very well at what times of the day you should eat which quantities of food and it is still highly topical. Especially if you have a damaged intestine, you should stick to it. Early in the morning and also at noon, the body needs energy to work, think and be active. There is still enough time before bedtime to digest the ingested food properly.

In the evening, the entire system slows down and prepares for the night. Heavy meals late at night then lie undigested in the stomach or in the intestine. During sleep, the body needs to recover and shuts down the digestive process.

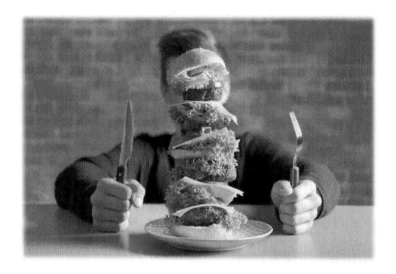

Therefore, portion sizes in the evening should be significantly smaller than at breakfast or lunch. Most important, the last meal should be eaten at least four hours before bedtime. For example, if you go to bed at 10 pm, your evening meal should be finished by 6 pm.

That is the theory. However, many people aren't hungry in the morning and for them, dinner is the best meal of the day. In the evening, the day's work is done and you have time to sit together with your friends and family. There is nothing wrong with this and it would not make sense to force your body into totally different habits. However, if you have digestive problems, you just have to make sure that dinner won't be a huge portion eaten right before going to bed.

Superfoods

Superfoods are certain foods that supposed to have an incredibly great effect on your health. Even though a new "superfood" is discovered almost every month – there is no such thing as a superfood. As I have mentioned before, this is simply an invention of the food industry to offer people something new.

So far, goji berries, chia seeds or chlorella algae have been allowed to join the circle of superfoods. When you see a product that is labeled as "healthy" or even "super healthy," then you should become suspicious. An apple or a carrot aren´t labeled as "healthy," although they are.

There is no single food that is super healthy. What is healthy above all is more a varied diet and, in the case of histamine intolerance, the avoidance of foods you can't tolerate.

Whole grains and raw foods

In nutritional counseling, it is repeatedly emphasized how important whole grain products and raw foods are for a healthy diet. In principle, we can agree with this, but with one important restriction: Whole grains and raw foods are only good if they are tolerated well. As I have mentioned before, these tips only apply to people with a healthy intestine.

Especially with histamine problems, the entire digestive tract is constantly in turmoil anyway and it should not be burdened even more. Whole grains contain a significantly higher amount of **fiber.** Therefore, whole grain products have more nutrients and at the same time, they feed our good intestinal bacteria.

The disadvantage of whole grain products is that they are much more difficult to digest. Therefore, you should not simply follow the advice "whole grains are always good," but here you just have to see what your gut says and trust your own body feeling.

The same is true for any form of **raw food**. Raw food include all foods that have not been heated, such as lettuce, seeds, nuts or cabbage. The disadvantage of heating food is that certain vitamins and enzymes in the food are lost while they are much more present in raw foods. However, if you are struggling with digestive problems, then cooked food is usually the better choice, since the heat from cooking makes the food much easier to digest than it is in raw form.

Chew thoroughly and do not eat a mix of too many foods
If you've ever watched a cow graze, you understand what thorough chewing is. Generally, it is recommended that each bite should be chewed about 30 times to make it easier for the subsequent digestive organs. The finer the food that enters the body, the more the burden on the digestive tract is relieved.

Besides grinding the food, chewing has another great benefit, since it mixes the food with saliva. Saliva contains enzymes that already start to break down parts of the food.

Therefore, digestion does not begin just in the stomach; it already starts in the mouth by chewing.

Well, it can certainly be very tedious and annoying to really chew every bite 30 times. However, if you can improve from almost not chewing up to chewing food 15 times, that's already a huge help for the digestive system. Of course, intolerances won't go away just by chewing food well, but it's another important step on the road to recovery.

Another thing that you should avoid when you have an upset digestive tract is **eating a mix of too many things**. Eating this way makes it much more likely that one of the foods will cause digestive problems. Furthermore, the stomach and intestine also have a hard time with a wild mixture of foods within one meal. The meal should still be fun and varied, but a three- or even five-course meal with appetizers and desert is just too much of a good thing for an already battered intestine.

Furthermore, **spicy food** can also irritate the intestine. On the one hand, hot spices can release the histamine which is stored in the body. All substances that release the body's own histamine are called histamine liberators. With spicy food, there is a much more important factor: Histamine generally acts as an inflammation booster in the body. Therefore, it often happens that the intestine of someone with histamine intolerance is struggling with inflammation, and an inflamed intestine is not happy about spicy things at all.

After we have looked into some general lifestyle and eating rules, we will now go deeper into the topic of the diagnosis and treatment for histamine intolerance.

3 Diagnosis and treatment

In this section, we now turn to the most important topic: How do I determine whether I have histamine intolerance and how is it treated.

Unfortunately, there is no single lab value that tells you very clearly whether you have histamine intolerance or not. Other intolerances like lactose or gluten can be clearly diagnosed, but as we have seen before, histamine is always a little more complex and we have to look at more than one factor. Histamine intolerance consists of two components: How much histamine is released in the body on a daily basis, and how well it is broken down.

The best method to determine if you are suffering from histamine intolerance is going on an elimination diet. This method is currently superior to almost any laboratory test. To do this, you leave out histamine-containing foods for about two to three weeks, as best you can. Histamine cannot be avoided completely anyway, but you should particularly avoid foods with a lot of histamine for the duration of the elimination diet.

When you notice that avoiding histamine makes you feel much better and the symptoms improve, then it is quite likely that you have histamine intolerance. Now you can start to track down the cause of your intolerance.

On the other hand, if your symptoms do not improve despite the strict avoidance of histamine, then you very likely do not have histamine intolerance and your symptoms are probably caused by something else.

Laboratory values can be very helpful in the search for the cause of the histamine intolerance. However, you must be somewhat careful with interpreting them. Let's take a look at this using two sample patients. Person A has problems with histamine-containing foods and has his DAO value checked. It turns out that the value is much below the reference value.

Now person A knows that he produces too little of the enzyme DAO and therefore he cannot sufficiently break histamine down. Therefore, every meal containing too much histamine will lead to trouble, because the histamine is not broken down properly. The goal here would be for his body to start producing more DAO enzymes again.

Person B also has problems with histamine and also has the DAO value measured. However, the lab value is fine and it shows that his body produces sufficient DAO. Because of the good DAO value, person B would now conclude that there is no histamine intolerance present. However, further investigation reveals that the histamine problems only began when person B started taking certain medications on a regular basis.

Since person B is not necessarily dependent on the medications, they are omitted or replaced by others and the histamine complaints improve significantly. Person B was able to break down histamine well, which was shown by the good DAO value, but the medications were constantly releasing the body's own histamine. In addition to the histamine in food, the body's own histamine was released by the medication – and that was simply too much for his body.

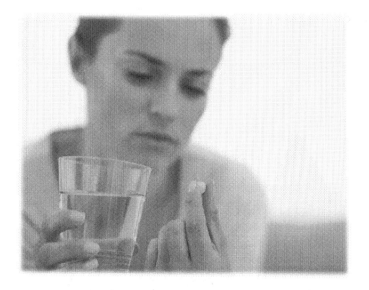

Based on these two examples, you can see that sometimes you have to look deeper to find the cause of the intolerance. In the following chapters, you will find the most common causes that can lead to histamine intolerance.

When you are completely new to the subject, then of course you can't test everything at once. That would be too much to ask and probably your piggy bank would go on strike as well. Therefore, it is important to have a plan for measuring what is most important and should come first. I have sorted out the chapters accordingly, starting with the most important measurements first. Other tests might come later, but only when the ones from the "very important category" are finished.

For example, it would make no sense to start with a genetical histamine test, which costs a lot of money. A genetic predisposition for histamine intolerance is very rare and there is not much you can do about it. This might be an option if you have already tried many other options before. Especially when you are at the beginning of testing and treatment, other measures would make much more sense like testing your DAO-enzyme value, a stool analysis or a heavy metal test.

As we have seen earlier, the long-term goal is to be cured of histamine intolerance instead of managing the symptoms. In order to do that, you need to get to the root causes and this takes time. As long as you still have problems with histamine, being careful of your diet is nothing additional, but rather is a very important part of the treatment.

If you eat whatever you feel like, the histamine overdose from food will increase the inflammatory processes in your body and your intestine will be stirred up by every meal. On the other hand, if a good diet goes hand in hand with a targeted treatment, then you have a good chance of recovering and your histamine intolerance may improve significantly or you may even say goodbye completely. Only if you consistently watch out for histamine in your diet and avoid it, will your body come to rest and your intestine is able to recover.

3.1   DAO enzyme – Our best friend in breaking down histamine

The term DAO does not mean "Danny Adores Oranges," but it rather describes the enzyme Di-Amin-Oxidase. This term is very important for everyone with histamine intolerance, since the DAO value shows how well histamine is broken down in the body.

More than 90% of this DAO enzyme is produced in the intestine [2]. Despite of this, DAO can be used everywhere in the body to break down histamine. Especially since DAO is produced almost exclusively in the small intestine, an important connection is immediately apparent: The worse the condition of the intestine, the less DAO is produced.

An ailing intestine includes disturbance of the bacterial flora, inflammatory processes (such as in Crohn's disease or ulcerative colitis) or it includes fungal infestation with candida fungi. The intestine is constantly exposed to threats and accordingly the reasons for an ailing intestine can be manifold.

How is DAO enzyme measured?

Since the DAO is not only supposed to act in the intestine, but is needed everywhere, it must be released into the blood so that it can subsequently be distributed throughout the body. That means that a good way for checking DAO is via a blood sample, but this value can fluctuate throughout the day. Therefore, it is recommended to have the value determined on two different days to obtain a more reliable result.

How to improve the DAO value?

If the measurement shows that your DAO value is too low, then the reason for your histamine intolerance has probably already been found. On the other hand, if your DAO value is not too low and it is within the standard range, then there must be another cause for the histamine problems. DAO is one reason, but there are many other reasons why histamine intolerance can arise.

The most common cause for a low DAO value is a **damaged gut**. In order to find out if this is the case for you, there are two possibilities. The first way is what you notice in your symptoms. If you frequently struggle with bloating, abdominal cramps, diarrhea or constipation, then this is already a first indication, that your intestine is not doing well.

However, you do not yet know what exactly is wrong in your intestine, but there is a very helpful and simple method to figure it out and that´s the stool sample. As we have seen before, there can be many causes behind a troubled intestine, be it an inflammation, candida fungi or problems with the intestinal bacteria.

The last thing you want to do is an anti-fungal treatment for half a year just on suspicion, even though you don't even have any intestinal fungi. In such a case, you have lost a lot of time, money and energy. As a result, you will be annoyed that the entire effort has been for nothing.

However, if you have a stool sample checked, you will know very precisely what is going on in your intestine and then you can take targeted action against it. We will deal with this important topic of the stool sample in more detail in *Chapter 3.3.*

Let´s get back to DAO enzyme. This is generally a very sensitive enzyme, because it does not occur inside the cells like most enzymes, but it must survive outside the cells, where it is exposed to many disruptive factors.

When the gut is weakened, then usually there is not enough DAO produced. This simply means that the amount of DAO is too low. However, it can also happen that the **amount of DAO** is high, but the DAO enzymes themselves are weak. Therefore, there are two decisive factors when it comes to DAO: The amount of it present as well as its activity level. The reason for this lack of DAO activity can be a **deficiency of certain vital nutrients** such as copper, zinc and vitamin B6.

A deficiency of these nutrients prevents the DAO from firing properly. This condition is called DAO activity disorder.

Furthermore, certain **drugs or alcohol** can block the activity of the DAO enzymes as well.

Overall, there can be three different ways in which the DAO enzyme no longer works properly:

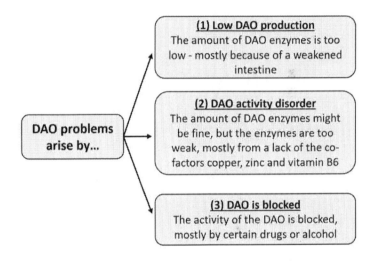

DAO problems arise by...

(1) Low DAO production
The amount of DAO enzymes is too low - mostly because of a weakened intestine

(2) DAO activity disorder
The amount of DAO enzymes might be fine, but the enzymes are too weak, mostly from a lack of the co-factors copper, zinc and vitamin B6

(3) DAO is blocked
The activity of the DAO is blocked, mostly by certain drugs or alcohol

Let's imagine that DAO enzyme is something like a vacuum cleaner and its job is to absorb the histamine in the body. The vacuum cleaner switch that you use to set the suction power corresponds to DAO production (low DAO production). When the intestine is healthy and can produce a lot of DAO enzyme, then this is as if you have turned the power switch all the way up.

However, the vacuum cleaner cannot work on its own yet. You must activate it by plugging it into the power supply.

Only with this energy can the components become active and do their work (DAO activity disorder). If it isn't plugged into the power, nothing works and this is exactly how the DAO must be activated.

Now you can happily vacuum away and spruce up your apartment since your vacuum cleaner is working splendidly. However, suddenly a sock gets caught in the front of the nozzle and you can´t vacuum anymore. This sock blocks everything, and this corresponds to a drug or to alcohol which blocks the DAO activity. In this case, all the components of the vacuum cleaner are working fine, it is turned on by the power connection, and yet something is blocking the whole process (DAO is blocked).

We can already see that DAO enzyme can be up against many obstacles. When vacuuming, we can easily fix the problem, because we see the blocking sock or we notice that the vacuum cleaner is not plugged into the power yet. The processes in our body are not so easy to see, but fortunately, modern laboratories can help us to uncover each single problem.

Info-Box

✓ DAO is the most important enzyme in the body for breaking down histamine

✓ More than 90% of the DAO is produced in the intestine

✓ The DAO value can be easily checked by a blood test

✓ A deficiency of certain nutrients (copper, zinc and vitamin B6) can limit the activity of DAO

✓ Certain drugs and alcohol can also block the activity of DAO

3.2 HNMT – Another enzyme for histamine degradation?

The constant use of technical terms on the subject of histamine can be quite annoying – and the next term is already waiting around the corner. Unfortunately, we can't just leave these terms out, because knowing them is the only way to request the right tests at the lab. Furthermore, it is only by using these terms that it becomes clear what exactly is meant, for example when you exchange information with other people who also suffer from histamine intolerance.

Let´s get on to it – the name of the enzyme HNMT is also extremely unwieldy when it is spelled out: Histamine N-Methyl-Transferase. Luckily, we can just stick with the abbreviation HNMT. In short, HNMT is an enzyme that also breaks down histamine.

We have already seen that the DAO enzyme helps us to break down histamine in the body. However, DAO can only break down free histamine outside the cells. If histamine is inside a cell, then the HNMT enzyme takes care of it.

Whether degradation goes on inside or outside a cell sounds somehow quite abstract. The best way to illustrate the whole process is to take a look at blood cells. The blood cells float around in the blood like small particles. If histamine now has to be broken down inside the blood cells, then HNMT takes care of it.

The remaining histamine in the blood stream is broken down by DAO enzyme. DAO enzyme itself does not enter the cells and cannot break down histamine inside them. That is why there are these two different degradation pathways: Histamine breakdown takes place inside a cell via HNMT and outside the cells it is done by DAO enzyme.

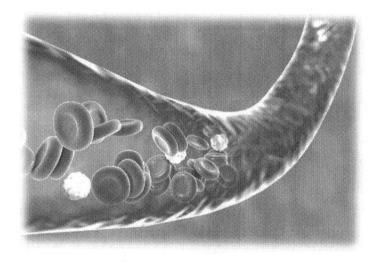

This spatial separation by the cells is important and it is also the reason why the two enzymes cannot replace each other. For example, if you have too few DAO enzymes, then HNMT cannot simply take over the DAO´s tasks. Due to the different modes of action, different symptoms arise. In the case of DAO deficiency, the body is not able to break down histamine from food properly. Therefore, histamine problems tend to occur in phases.

However, if there is not enough HNMT enzyme in the body, then the symptoms show up much more slowly and constantly. The problems therefore do not necessarily occur in conjunction with a meal. HNMT works primarily in the liver, kidney, bronchial tubes, brain and central nervous system. That is the reason why the typical symptoms of HNMT deficiency are restlessness, muscle twitching, sleep disturbances, fatigue, dizziness and anxiety.

DAO enzyme does not occur at all in the central nervous system. Here, histamine is only broken down by HNMT. This is the reason why the typical symptoms often occur in the area of the nerves in the case of HNMT weakness. HNMT weakness literally "gets on your nerves."

There are two reasons why the activity of HNMT enzyme is reduced. One of them may be a genetic defect, and there is not much that can be done about it. However, the lack of HNMT can also arise from certain environmental influences, and these are primarily drugs since they can suppress HNMT activity. We have already seen a similar effect with DAO enzyme, when drugs can inhibit the activity of the DAO enzymes.

If HNMT weakness is due to a medication, your histamine problems usually improve as soon as the medication is discontinued. However, it must first be clear that the histamine problems have arisen as a result of the medication and you cannot simply avoid or discontinue all medications. If the HNMT weakness is caused by medications, then you have a chance to do something about it. On the other hand, if it comes from a genetic defect, then improvement is much more difficult to achieve.

How can HNMT weakness be measured?
The amount of DAO enzyme can be determined very well by means of a blood test. For the HNMT enzyme, no such measurement is possible. You can´t determine whether someone is suffering from HNMT weakness or not just by means of a lab test.

Maybe it should be said that this is not possible **yet**, because laboratory medicine is developing very quickly and meanwhile it is already possible to determine countless parameters in the body – why not also HNMT one day?

However, there are genetic tests that can be used to check whether certain genes that are associated with HNMT are restricted in their function. One of them is the C314T genotype. However, the result of the genetic test does not say much about the HNMT itself. It only says that a certain gene does not function well and therefore HNMT weakness **could be** present, but that´s not for sure.

Imagine that your car won't start early in the morning. The repair shop could then read a single random value from the car's control unit, out of thousands of values that are stored there. You then have this value in black and white. However, it is completely unclear if it has anything to do with the actual problem. It would make much more sense for the repair shop to first check for much more obvious reasons. For example, they could test if the battery still has enough power or if the spark plugs are working fine.

Like the car, it works the same way with the HNMT genetic test. It would make much more sense to first check completely different causes for histamine intolerance before doing the HNMT genetic test. At the current state of science, the genetic test simply does not yet provide enough information that could really be useful for any treatment. Therefore, I would not recommend genetic testing for HNMT weakness at this time.

To summarize the topic of HNMT, it is important to know that HNMT enzyme is involved in the breakdown of histamine. And if you notice from your symptoms, that a HNMT weakness could be the reason, then you can do something about it, if the HNMT is caused by environmental influences or medications. Then it will even be possible to get a HNMT weakness back under control.

Although DAO enzyme and HNMT enzyme both break down histamine in the body, there are some differences between them:

	DAO enzyme	HNMT enzyme
Task	Histamine breakdown	Histamine breakdown
Place of activity	Outside the cells (extracellular)	Inside the cells (intracellular)
Symptoms when too low	>> Symptoms occur intermittently, depending on what was eaten >> They can occur almost anywhere	>> Rather constant symptoms >> Independent of food >> Symptoms mainly in the area of nerves
How can you test for it?	The amount of DAO enzyme can be determined by a blood sample – but the activity of DAO is usually not measured	Not measurable; genetic tests have little significance and are expensive
Why could this enzyme be too low?	Intestinal problems, hormonal imbalances, alcohol, medications	Medications or a genetic disorder

3.3 How is your intestine doing?

As we have seen, over 90% of DAO enzyme is produced in the intestine. When the intestine is in a bad state and produces too little DAO enzymes, then histamine in the body can no longer be broken down properly. Therefore, the intestine is a central starting point in case of histamine intolerance.

Our intestine is exposed to constant threats like viruses, bacteria, worms, fungi or other parasites. The intestine can also suffer from inflammation or it can become permeable (leaky gut syndrome). Furthermore, there can be a small intestinal bacterial overgrowth (SIBO), when the bacteria have migrated from the large intestine to the small intestine.

As if all this were not enough, our intestine faces another major disadvantage: It is the last link in the digestive chain. When we eat something, the first step of digestion begins directly in the mouth. After that comes the stomach, the gall bladder and then the pancreas.

If one of these digestive organs no longer does its job properly, then the food is not digested well and it reaches the intestine in a far too coarse form. The poorly digested food then lies in the intestine for a long time, begins to ferment and thus particularly harmful intestinal bacteria can spread easily.

It is therefore important that all digestive organs function well. A common reason why the **stomach** fails in the digestive chain is the use of so-called proton pump inhibitors (PPIs). These drugs are colloquially known as gastric acid blockers. Doctors prescribe these medicines usually against frequent heartburn and they reduce the production of gastric acid almost completely to zero.

However, if the stomach no longer produces gastric acid, this has several serious consequences. On the one hand, the extremely acidic gastric juice can no longer support digestion. You probably suspect already who has to pay for this in the end ... of course, it is our intestine! The intestine relies on the stomach to do a thorough preliminary job, because otherwise it has to do twice the work – its own job and the missing work by the stomach.

There is also a second disadvantage of these stomach acid blockers. Normally, certain invaders like bacteria, viruses or fungi have no chance of surviving in the stomach acid. The stomach acid acts like a gatekeeper who lets the good food pass and fights the bad invaders.

If you hardly produce any stomach acid due to taking these stomach acid blockers, then intruders have an easy time. Now they can slip past the gatekeeper and make themselves at home in the intestine.

And there is a third problem that comes up by the use of gastric acid blockers. The pancreas does not produce its secretion all day long. It only becomes active when it receives the signal "*Here comes food,*" and this signal comes from the stomach acid due to its acidic pH value. So, if there is a lack of stomach acid, the pancreas no longer works properly either, because its signal transmitter is missing.

It sounds simple to just take a small pill to deal with stomach acid problems and heartburn. However, "only" taking a gastric acid blocker can have very far-reaching consequences for the intestine and the bacterial flora. From this example of stomach acid blockers, we can see the far-reaching consequences that medications can have, especially when they are taken over a longer period of time.

This example demonstrates the basic principle that everything is interrelated in the body. Whenever you change one thing, it will have an effect on something else. Even if you just take a "little" pill regularly, it will have side effects, especially since the histamine balance in the body is very sensitive.

When we take a closer look at our intestine, we see that it is an incredibly fascinating organ. It is around six meters long, houses over 80% of our entire immune system, and it is home to several million nerve cells and therefore is also called the second brain. It produces over 90% of the DAO enzyme as well as other digestive enzymes, for example to break down lactose and fructose. The intestine is therefore highly complex, but also highly sensitive to external influences.

Many different processes interlock in the intestine and meanwhile it is constantly exposed to various attacks. This is exactly the reason why so many people suffer from intestinal problems. The intestine is highly complex and at the same time it is very sensitive to external influences.

However, there is also good news: You can do a lot to support your intestine. There are thousands of remedies that can be helpful for the intestine, but you don't want to try them all one after another.

Therefore, you first have to see what is not going well in your intestine and then you can take targeted action against this problem. This procedure should be followed with every disease: First check and measure what is wrong – that's the **diagnosis part,** and only when you know exactly where the problem lies, then the **treatment** takes place.

How to measure the health of the intestine?
When the intestine is not well, it shows its discomfort through symptoms such as flatulence, abdominal pain, cramps, diarrhea, constipation or histamine problems. Unfortunately, the intestine does not tell us what exactly is wrong, because it doesn't speak in words.

That is why we need another way to communicate with it to find the cause of these problems. In order to do that, we can take advantage of the very latest scientific laboratory tests. Just from a small sample of blood, stool or urine, incredible amounts of analysis can be done these days.

I am working as a scientist in a hospital and I am in regular touch with different laboratories. It is amazing to see how quickly laboratory medicine is developing; we are no longer talking about 20 or 30 different values that can be analyzed in total. Nowadays, several thousand parameters can be checked. And it is not the case that the result might be correct or maybe not: Instead, modern laboratory measurements are extremely reliable.

For histamine intolerance, we will take advantage of this very advanced laboratory measurements which are available to us. Specifically for the bowel and digestive problems in general, a stool sample is a great way to see where the problem comes from.

You can have this stool sample analysis done by a doctor or an alternative practitioner. In the following, I have compiled all the values that I would recommend for a stool sample. Most laboratories are very flexible when you order certain tests. Mostly, you will find a "standard profile" with certain values, but you can add more values you want to be checked.

For the stool sample, it is very important to have many values measured at once and not just one or two individual values. If you leave something out, then it may be exactly this value which provides the solution for your intestinal and histamine problems. The whole puzzle can only be put together by taking all these values together.

For a complete stool sample, I would recommend measuring these values:

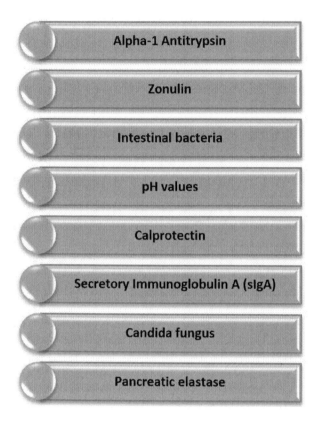

- Alpha-1 Antitrypsin
- Zonulin
- Intestinal bacteria
- pH values
- Calprotectin
- Secretory Immunoglobulin A (sIgA)
- Candida fungus
- Pancreatic elastase

Let's take a closer look at each single value. However, I have to warn you that there are some real tongue twisters in there, since laboratories mostly use a very cryptic language.

To determine if an **inflammation is** present in the intestine, you must look at the calprotectin level as well as alpha-1 antitrypsin. Inflammations are mostly a defense reaction and can occur almost anywhere in the body. They are usually accompanied by redness and warmth.

Furthermore, inflamed areas get more blood flow, which means they get more oxygen and nutrients. In addition, toxins are removed more quickly and the heat helps in the fight against invaders. That means, an inflammation that lasts a short time is something very helpful, while an inflammation that lasts a long time is a sign that something is out of balance.

Furthermore, a stool sample can be used to analyze the **intestinal bacteria**. There are well over 1,000 different species of intestinal bacteria in our intestine. The largest species are the bifidobacteria and the lactobacilli. These two species are checked in most cases during a stool examination.

With the values **zonulin** and **alpha-1 antitrypsin,** you can see if the intestine has become permeable. This condition is called "leaky gut syndrome." Normally, the cells in the intestine are firmly connected to each other. However, there are certain events during which the body expands these cell connections on purpose in order to obtain energy very quickly. In this way, it prepares itself for a possible escape or an attack, when large amounts of energy are needed very quickly.

However, various influences can cause the intestine to become permanently permeable. As a result, food components, toxins and harmful substances can slip through uncontrollably.

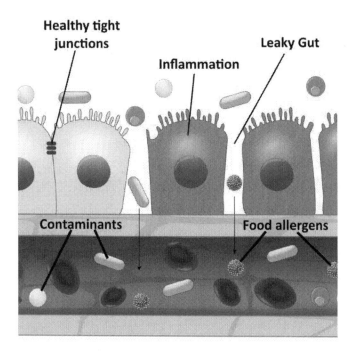

Another value in the stool sample is the **pH value.** It indicates whether the environment in the intestine is more acidic or alkaline. However, the stool sample only measures the pH value of the intestine and not the pH value of the entire body, which is determined from the urine. The ideal pH value of the intestine is between 5.8 and 6.5. At a pH value above

6.5, the "bad" intestinal bacteria feel very comfortable and spread significantly faster.

To see how active the immune system in the intestine is, the value **secretory immunoglobulin A (sIgA)** can be measured. This value can swing upwards or downwards, and that means that the immune system in the intestine is either too weak or it is excessively active. Another reason for a high sIgA value can be that an inflammation is present in the intestine.

Our intestine is constantly exposed to a wide variety of attackers. Since there are countless types of viruses, bacteria or fungi, it is not possible to measure them all with a stool sample. However, there are some usual suspects that often are present in connection with digestive problems and this includes **candida yeast fungus** in particular.

When the intestinal flora is out of balance, for example after taking antibiotics, then these candida fungi find excellent conditions to spread and they particularly like to feed on sugars and white flour products.

The candida fungus is quite a stubborn fellow, as it clings to the surface of the intestine and can even survive longer periods of starvation. If you radically deprive it of food, then it bores even deeper into the intestinal mucosa in order to reach food via the blood. This is the reasons why you should never starve out a candida fungus. You won´t get rid of it and instead, the fungal infestation only gets worse.

The last important laboratory value in our bundle is the **pancreatic elastase**. This value has nothing to do directly with the intestine, but measures the activity of the pancreas. Simply said, it looks at how much juice the pancreas is releasing.

The pancreas produces digestive juices for breaking down protein, carbohydrates and fats. The performance of the pancreas is very important for the intestine, because the pancreas is part of the digestive chain and it is located ahead of the intestine in this chain. When the pancreas does not function properly, the intestine has to take the brunt and is eventually overwhelmed with this extra work.

When we are talking about weakness of the pancreas, this should not be mixed up with pancreatitis. A weak pancreas is nothing dramatic and does not mean that something is seriously wrong with your pancreas. It only means that the pancreas is no longer working at full capacity and should be brought back up to speed.

Even if we devote ourselves very intensively to the intestine in this chapter, this still leads us back to the topic of histamine intolerance. The intestine is the decisive degradation center for histamine, since 90% of the histamine-eating DAO enzyme is formed here. An ailing intestine and histamine intolerance are closely linked to each other.

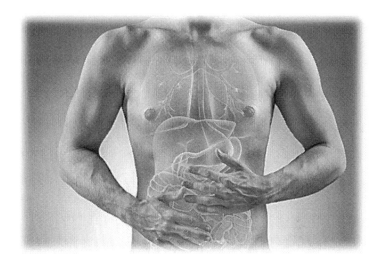

To get all the laboratory values that I have mentioned above, you don´t have to measure every value on its own. All values can be determined from only one single stool sample. This could hardly be more convenient and instructions are provided for each stool sample set, so it is almost impossible for you to do anything wrong.

What can be done to deal with intestinal problems?

If you suffer from digestive problems, then of course you want to get started immediately and do something about them. However, since there are thousands of remedies that could help, it's like the famous search for the needle in a haystack. That is exactly the reason why it is so important to take a stool sample first, so that you know exactly how you should proceed.

1) Remedies against inflammation

When the levels of calprotectin and alpha-1 antitrypsin are elevated, the intestine is currently struggling with an inflammation. It is good to know if there is an inflammation or not, but that's just one part of the journey. The next step is to find out why there is an inflammation present, since there can be multiple reasons for that.

One very helpful function of histamine in the body is to initiate an inflammation or maintain an existing inflammation. If too much histamine is buzzing uncontrollably through the body, as it is the case with histamine intolerance, then this excess histamine can lead to a permanent inflammation. Since food is primarily broken down in the intestine, an overdose of histamine is particularly present in the intestine.

In case of an intestinal inflammation, the primary goal is to gradually rebuild the intestine: Via having good intestinal bacteria, avoiding foods you can't tolerate, less stress, regular meals and generally a healthy lifestyle.

A particularly good remedy against inflammation is **vitamin C**, which can be given either as a dietary supplement or by a therapist as a high-dose infusion. **Zinc, amino acids, Omega-3 fatty acids and bone broth** have also proven effective. Among all amino acids, **L-glutamine** is particularly noteworthy against digestive problems. The rapidly dividing cells in the intestine are very fond of L-glutamine, as they can use it excellently as a building material.

Since most people with intestinal and histamine problems do not tolerate many dietary supplements, infusions are a good alternative. Amino acids in particular, which are a proven remedy against inflammation, are tolerated much better by most patients in the form of an infusion. Some manufacturers even have ready-made infusion mixtures that are specially adapted for food intolerances.

Another reason for an inflammation in the intestine can be viruses, worms or other parasites. However, since there are many different invaders, they cannot be measured with a single test. We will take a closer look at the most important intruders later.

2) Leaky gut – The permeable bowel
If the stool sample has shown that the zonulin or alpha-1 antitrypsin levels are elevated, then you are probably dealing with a leaky gut.

The intestine becomes permeable when the cell connections no longer lie firmly close together. These cell connections are also called "tight junctions." There can be several causes for the intestine to become permeable. One reason for this may be an inflammation. If the inflammation is controlled, the leaky gut syndrome usually disappears.

However, stress can also lead to leaky gut syndrome. The body has learned over millennia that there are moments when it must immediately flee or attack. For these extreme situations, it needs energy. In fact, it needs a lot of energy and preferably as quickly as possible.

It cannot wait until the food has been completely digested in the intestine. Instead, it opens the cell connections in order to access the energy reserves very quickly. Once that extreme situation is over, the cell connections are firmly closed again.

However, through permanent and intense stress, the body is led to believe that the escape or attack situation still exists. Thus, the cell connections in the intestine will remain opened and a leaky gut syndrome develops.

A third reason for a leaky gut is an imbalance of the intestinal gut flora. When there are just too many bad bacteria, then toxins arise, the mucous membrane can't build up properly or an inflammation can develop. Therefore, a bacterial imbalance can also be a reason for developing leaky gut.

3) Intestinal bacteria

Besides the lab values already mentioned, the intestinal flora can also be analyzed precisely from a stool sample. For this purpose, the number of *bifidobacteria* and *lactobacilli* is usually measured. If it turns out that there are too few good intestinal bacteria, then there are very helpful remedies to get things back in balance. One of the most effective ways is consuming products that contain good intestinal bacteria.

Normally, a reliable and inexpensive method to get good bacteria is to eat sauerkraut as well as pickled vegetables. However, for anyone with a histamine intolerance, this should be avoided, since these foods contain a lot of histamine. If you eat sauerkraut or pickled vegetables despite your histamine intolerance, then it does more harm than good.

When the intestinal flora is out of balance, then the intestine can no longer properly perform its tasks. Digestion no longer functions well and an inflammation can occur. All this puts a lot of strain on the intestine and the more it is burdened, the worse is it able to take care of producing the important DAO enzyme.

To make matters worse, there are certain strains of bacteria that produce histamine on their own. This is of course extremely unfavorable in case of histamine intolerance. Therefore, such intestinal bacteria products (called probiotics) should be carefully selected, so that they are well tolerated. You will usually notice pretty quickly if you can't tolerate a gut bacteria product and in that case, you should not use it anymore.

Bacterial species that produce tyramine are also unsuitable when you have a histamine intolerance. This is because tyramine is a biogenic amine just like histamine. The DAO enzyme preferentially breaks down tyramine first and the more DAO is used for tyramine, the less is left for the breakdown of histamine.

However, so that you don't have to examine every gut bacteria product for all the individual bacteria strains, there are some probiotics that are specifically made for people with a histamine intolerance. In these products, the bacterial species and further ingredients are selected with the focus to histamine intolerant patients.

Strains of bacteria that do NOT produce histamine or tyramine
ALL bifidobacteria (large intestine)
Lactobacillus gasseri (small intestine)
Lactobacillus rhamnosus (small intestine)
Lactobacillus salivarius (small intestine)
Lactobacillus sporogenes (small intestine)
Lactobacillus plantarum (small intestine)

Table 1: Bacterial species that do not produce histamine or tyramine [7].

4) Viruses, bacteria, fungi and worms

Our body is constantly threatened by many attackers. It is not so easy for the attackers to enter the body through the skin, but they can enter the body much more easily by food or water.

You usually know that you have acute gastrointestinal flu due to severe symptoms such as diarrhea or vomiting. The doctor can identify certain diseases by such symptoms and they usually disappear after a few days. However, what if an invader has taken up residence in the intestine for a longer period of time and won´t go on its own? To check this, the doctor can look for specific attackers by taking a blood sample as well as a stool sample. The most well-known species associated with intestinal problems include:

Viruses
such as adeno- ,astro-, rota- or norovirus

Bacteria
such as campylobacter, salmonella, shigella or yersinia

Protozoans
such as amoebas, lamblia or cryptosporidium

Worms
and worm eggs

Fungi
such as candida

As you can see, the human body is exposed to many attackers. The best place to get a comprehensive test, which checks for as many invaders as possible, is from a gastroenterologist or from a general practitioner. The whole process of checking for an intruder is very simple for patients: You just give a blood or stool sample and a few days later you will get the results.

Normally, health insurance companies pay for the examination for a large number of known attackers. However, there must always be a reasonable suspicion of their presence and some doctors are a bit more hesitant. If your doctor does not want to perform this examination for you, then you always have the right to see another doctor.

If the findings are indeed abnormal, then the doctor will decide what to do next. However, it may well be that your treatment is successful, but your histamine and abdominal complaints still do not improve. This is not at all uncommon and means that this specific intruder was not the real cause for your histamine intolerance. It is good to get rid of it, but then you have to keep looking for the actual cause of the histamine intolerance.

I also have been checked for the most important viruses, bacteria and worms and something was found – it was a small, nice Giardia lamblia. This is a single-celled parasite, which is known that it likes to cause trouble in the gastrointestinal tract. I even had to report it to the health department, but mainly to prevent a major spread early on.

I probably brought this nice fellow back from my travels in India.

The doctor then treated the parasite with antibiotics and found after another stool sample it was no longer detectable. However, the digestive disorders didn´t improve after the treatment, which indicates that the Giardia lamblia was not the cause of my intestinal problems.

If nothing abnormal is found in such a test, then at least you have clarity and you are again able to exclude a source of danger from the list. However, in case something is found, then you have the chance to take concrete action against this parasite.

5) The intestinal immune system
With a stool sample, you can not only test for an inflammation or the number of intestinal bacteria, but you can even check the condition of your immune system in the intestine. This is done by means of the "secretory immunoglobulin A" (sIgA) value.

This value can deviate into two directions: Either it is too low or too high. If the value is too high, your immune system in the intestine is very active at the moment. This could mean that there is an inflammation or the intestine is dealing with pathogens. Since one of the main tasks of the immunoglobulins is to defend against enemies, it becomes highly active when it has to fight certain pathogens.

Thus, if the sIgA level is elevated, it is worth while taking further tests for viruses, bacteria and parasites. On the other hand, if there is an inflammation in the intestine, the sIgA level may return to normal as soon as the inflammation has subsided.

The other possibility is that the sIgA value is too low and this means that the immune system in the intestine is usually weakened and should be revived. All measures that are generally good for the immune system can help here: Plenty of fresh air, sufficient exercise, lots of fresh fruit and vegetables (if tolerated) or sauna sessions.

A supplement to help get the immune system well back on track is **colostrum**. It is the first milk of mammals immediately after giving birth. In the commercially available products, the colostrum from cows is often used.

After birth, the newborn's immune system is quite weak, as it was protected by the mother's immune system the whole time in the womb. Therefore, the first milk contains a particularly high number of ingredients that are specifically needed to strengthen the immune system. That's why colostrum contains a lot of vitamins, minerals and trace elements. But above all, it consists of natural immune stimulating factors as well as important amino acids.

If you are lactose intolerant, there are also lactose-free colostrum products. However, colostrum might cause problems for someone with histamine intolerance. This also depends somewhat on the personal tolerance as well as on the colostrum product itself and must simply be tested.

Info-Box

✓ Since 90% of DAO enzyme is produced in the gut, intestinal health is an important factor in histamine intolerance

✓ Many things can be out of whack in the gut: The intestinal flora, the pH level, candida fungi, inflammation or the intestine may have become permeable (leaky gut)

✓ A stool sample can be used to scientifically and reliably determine what is causing problems in the intestine

✓ Depending on your own, individual result of the stool sample, concrete action can than be taken against these problems

3.4 Vitamin and mineral deficiencies

As we have seen, more than 90% of DAO enzyme is produced in the small intestine. However, this does not mean that this DAO enzyme can become **active** in the body. This is similar to when you are using a vacuum cleaner. You want to start vacuuming, the vacuum cleaner is fully assembled and all components are working. However, as long as there is no electricity, it simply won´t work. The same is true for DAO enzyme: Even if enough amount of DAO enzymes is being produced, as long as certain substances are missing, the DAO cannot become properly active.

These substances that contribute to activating the DAO enzyme are called co-factors. First and foremost, these include **copper, zinc and vitamin B6**. Also important for good DAO production, but not of the highest priority, are vitamin C, manganese, calcium and magnesium [9].

If not enough DAO enzymes are produced in the intestine due to the intestinal problems, then we speak of a **DAO deficiency**. In this case, there is simply not enough DAO enzyme to completely break down the histamine which is produced daily. However, if enough DAO is produced, but it cannot become properly active, then we speak of a **DAO activity disorder**. At this point, we come to a major problem when talking about DAO in the context of histamine intolerance.

The DAO value can be measured via blood, but here you have to be careful: The laboratory test only measures the amount of DAO. If your DAO value is fine, then in most cases, this only means that you produce enough DAO enzyme. However, this says nothing about how powerful or how active the DAO really is.

Until 2012, there was only one test for DAO enzyme. This test was very difficult for the laboratories to perform, since it involved radioactive radiation and working with radioactive material requires a lot of additional cost and work for a lab. However, with this test, it was possible to measure the amount of DAO as well as its activity level.

Since 2012, there has been an ELISA test for DAO, which is much easier for the labs to perform. The disadvantage of this test is that it only measures the amount of DAO, but it does NOT measure its activity. In the laboratory results, both the amount as well as the activity are stated in units per liter (U/l) and this makes it hard for patients to recognize what exactly was measured.

The only way to get to know what exactly was measured (the amount or activity), is to check with the lab. In the vast majority of cases, only the amount of DAO is measured and you will not get any information about the activity of your DAO. However, there are some indications that point to a significant reduction in activity and these mainly include the co-factors.

The current levels of copper, zinc and vitamin B6 can be determined via the blood. However, it is essential to have these values measured in the **whole blood** instead of just the serum. For the patient, this makes no difference at all and only a small blood sample is taken for both cases. The difference is, that in the serum test only minerals and vitamins which are freely present in the blood are measured. On the other hand, measuring them in the whole blood shows how much of the measured vitamins and minerals are stored inside the cells [10].

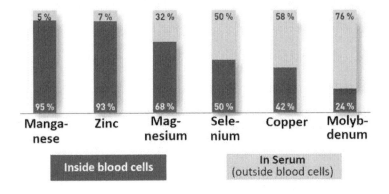

Figure 1: Distribution of minerals inside vs. outside of cells [10]

When you test in whole blood, you can see the overall status of your vitamins and minerals in extracellular (outside the cells) and intracellular (inside the cells). The graph above shows for example, that over 42% of copper and even 93% of zinc is stored inside the blood cells.

If you have the test performed using blood serum, only a certain portion of these minerals and vitamins will be measured and thus no reliable results would be obtained. In most cases, you have to actively request a measurement in whole blood from your doctor, because health insurance companies often will only pay for a test measuring these elements in the serum.

The reasons for a lack of nutrients can be quite different. One reason is malnutrition, when unhealthy foods low in nutrients are frequently consumed or when there is almost no variety in the diet. Another reason for a deficiency of

86

nutrients can be a weakly functioning pancreas or intestinal problems. In such a case, even if you have sufficient intake of minerals and vitamins, it might not be absorbed into the body. This means, if the digestive organs do not function optimally, this usually leads to significantly lower nutrient absorption.

However, there is also a third possibility for a lack of nutrients. This is the case, when sufficient nutrients are taken in and they are absorbed well, but at the same time the body consumes too many nutrients. This is especially the case with intensive sports or permanent stress.

There are quite a few reasons why certain nutrients might be lacking. Vitamins and minerals do not occur in the body by the kilogram; they are present only in very small quantities. However, even if only a few milligrams of certain vitamins or minerals are missing, this can already have serious consequences and lead to diseases.

In the following, we take a closer look at the three most important co-factors for the DAO enzyme – copper, zinc and vitamin B6.

Copper

Copper is one of the trace elements and is essential for us, since the body cannot produce it by itself. About 70 - 150 mg of copper are stored in the body.

Currently, there are 16 enzymes known in which copper is involved. In addition to DAO, they also include superoxide dismutase (SOD), which protects the cell membrane from free radicals and is thus an antioxidant. Furthermore, copper is involved in the energy production as well as blood formation. It is also needed for forming melanin in the skin, which works to improve the immune system and fight inflammation [11].

For most healthy people, copper is not considered a critical trace element. However, for someone with digestive disorders, a lack of copper is very likely, because the body heavily consumes copper, especially during an inflammation.

The main sources of copper are liver (especially calf's liver), fish, shellfish, nuts and cocoa as well as some green vegetables. However, people with histamine intolerance aren't able to tolerate many of these foods.

As a result, you can´t eat copper-rich foods because of your histamine intolerance. In addition, when the intestine is damaged, not enough copper is absorbed. This is also the case for many other nutrients. Therefore, replenishing copper reserves through diet alone is difficult and dietary supplements can do a good job here.

Zinc

As we have seen, copper is already involved in the formation of over 16 enzymes. However, zinc clearly outperforms copper, since more than 100 enzymes contain zinc or they are activated by zinc [12]. So, the dependence of our DAO enzyme on zinc is not at all rare among enzymes.

In addition to playing a key role in enzymes, zinc is important for wound healing. That's why many wound healing creams are enriched with zinc. Furthermore, zinc protects the organism from damage by oxygen radicals; it is essential for the development and function of the immune system and the excretion of carbon dioxide via the lungs would not be possible without zinc [12].

When absorbed into the body, zinc competes with other minerals such as calcium, iron, selenium and copper. Therefore, supplements containing iron or copper should not be taken at the same time as zinc supplements.

If you want to increase your zinc level using dietary supplements, then the supplement's chemical composition plays an important role. To understand this, you don't have to take a chemistry course. All you have to do is to look at the ingredients list and see which word follows the zinc, for example, zinc gluconate or zinc picolinate.

This tells you what chemical compound of zinc it contains. The zinc compound is important, because the body can absorb some zinc compounds very well, while others are not well absorbed.

Manufacturers like to use zinc gluconate or orotate, since they are inexpensive. However, the body absorbs these zinc compounds quite poorly. On the other hand, zinc picolinate or zinc chelates are much easier for the body to absorb.

Vitamin B6

For anyone with histamine intolerance, a vitamin B6 deficiency is not unlikely. The intestine is not working that well compared to healthy people and therefore significantly less vitamin B6 is absorbed. In addition to the lack of absorption, the diet is significantly more restricted than for people who aren't histamine intolerant.

Besides this, there are even more reasons for an increased need for Vitamin B6. These include taking hormonal contraceptives, eating disorders, the use of certain medications such as antidepressants or anticonvulsants and a high alcohol consumption. The reasons for a deficiency of vitamin B6 are manifold.

The major tasks of vitamin B6 is to convert amino acids; it plays a crucial role in the formation of hemoglobin (red blood cells) and bile acid. It also contributes to strengthening the nervous system and strengthening the immune system. Vitamin B6 is involved in the production of many hormones and it also has an enormously important function for enzymes: Without a sufficient supply of vitamin B6, up to 100 enzymes in the body cannot function properly.

Vitamin B6 can exist in three different chemical compounds in food: As pyridoxine, pyridoxal and pyridoxamine (don´t worry, you don´t have to remember them). However, the body always has to convert these three original (inactive) forms into active vitamin B6. Only then it can be used in the body. This active form is called pyridoxal-5-phosphate, also known as **P-5-P**.

If you want to improve your vitamin B6 level by taking dietary supplements, it is important to choose a product that already contains the active form. This is easy to recognize, because the term "P-5-P" should be written on the label. When you take vitamin B6 in form of P-5-P, your body can absorb much more of it. The body doesn´t have to go a long way to convert the vitamin into its active form itself, since it is already available in the activated form.

Importance for histamine intolerance	Nutrient	Recommended intake for adults per day	
		Men	Women
Very important	Copper	1.0–1.5 mg	1.0–1.5 mg
	Zinc	14 mg	8 mg
	Vitamin B6	1.6 mg	1.4 mg
Important	Vitamin C	110 mg	95 mg
	Magnesium	350-400 mg	300-310 mg
	Calcium	1000 mg	1000 mg
	Manganese	2–5 mg	2–5 mg

Table 2: Nutrients and vitamins that are important in case of histamine intolerance – reference values according to the recommendations of the German Society for Nutrition [13].

Although the reference values you can see in the table are good indication, they are only average values. An athlete or construction worker probably need a completely different consumption than an office worker does. Based on the recommended values, you can only see which quantities an average person should consume per day. And the recommended values do not say anything about how much is actually absorbed by the body.

Let's assume that a healthy person eats a banana containing 50 mg of magnesium and absorbs about 45 mg of magnesium, since a certain amount is always lost. Someone else who has intestinal problems absorbs only 20 mg from the same banana, because the intestine simply cannot absorb nutrients very well.

Theoretically, both people have consumed 50 mg of magnesium by eating one banana, but the amounts that arrive in the body are totally different. That's the reason why reference values help as a good point of orientation, but they say nothing about how much of the consumed amount the body can actually use.

Some people think: "*Ohh, minerals and vitamins are in general crucial for my health and I need to supplement them as much as I can.*" That is for sure the wrong way. You might supplement certain nutrients that you are not low on at all, and you might forget nutrients that you are really lacking.

Even for healthy people, it is important to be well supplied with vitamins and minerals, since they are important for many processes in our body. And as we have seen before, especially for someone with histamine intolerance, a deficiency can be the cause for many digestive symptoms.

Before supplementing anything, you need to figure out if you have a deficiency of certain nutrients or if you are well supplied. There is a very simple and reliable way to do that – you have to measure the levels first by means of laboratory values. Only then can you see whether a major deficiency has developed over time or if everything is fine and a deficiency can even occur despite of good nutrition.

To make this very concrete, a nutrient analysis would proceed as follows: You go to a doctor or alternative practitioner and determine which values should be measured. In case of histamine intolerance, the minimum is to check for copper, zinc, vitamin B6, magnesium, calcium and vitamin C. Then the blood sample is sent to a laboratory and some days later, the doctor gets the results back.

However, if you get a nutrient analysis done, I would recommend **measuring as many nutrients and vitamins as possible**. This gives you a complete overview and you won't miss anything. I would recommend testing for:

Chromium	Vitamin A
Manganese	Vitamin C
Sodium	Vitamin E
Calium	Vitamin D (25 OH)
Magnesium	Vitamin K
Calcium	Vitamin B1
Copper	Vitamin B2
Iron	Vitamin B3
Zinc	Vitamin B6
Selenium	Vitamin B12
Biotin	Coenzym Q10
Folic acid	

Especially vitamin D and vitamin B12 are also very important in context of histamine intolerance and for overall health as well.

And as we remember: No matter which vitamins and minerals you get measured – it is very important to get them tested in the **whole blood**. Most likely, you have to ask your therapist to test the nutrients in whole blood instead in serum. When checking nutrients just in serum, you only get to see how many of them are stored outside the blood cells. However, testing nutrients in whole blood is the only way to see how many of the nutrient are actually stored outside as well as inside the cells.

The laboratory result can then be used to identify which nutrients are present in sufficient quantities and where improvement is needed. Supplements should only be taken in consultation with a therapist and, of course, a healthy and balanced diet is always the foundation.

Without a balanced diet, it will not take long until you have a deficiency again. The supplements are in no way intended to be taken permanently. They should only be used to boost you out of the deficiency.

After a few months of topping up your nutrients, you can then take another laboratory test. In this second test, you only need to measure the values that were conspicuously low before and see if your supplemental therapy was already successful.

Info-Box

✓ To be fully efficient and activated, the DAO enzyme needs the nutrients copper, zinc and vitamin B6 – they are so called co-factors of DAO

✓ The nutrients should be measured in whole blood and not only in serum

✓ For a good and comprehensive analysis, other values should also be checked in order to get a complete picture of your current mineral and vitamin status

3.5   Heavy metals and the myth of amalgam

Based on this discussion about nutrients, we have seen how sensitive the body is and that missing substances even in a very small amount can already have major effects. Just as the absence of certain good substances can trigger an illness, too many toxins can lead to health problems as well.

In recent years, heavy metals in particular have stood out among the toxic substances that can lead to development of diseases. There are many reports of sufferers with intestinal problems who were able to make significant progress or even got completely rid of their disease by eliminating heavy metals.

Of course, this does not mean that you have half a kilogram of lead in your intestine and therefore your digestion is not running smoothly. The amount that can make you sick is only in the milligram range and yet even this small amount can have enormous effects on your health.

The tricky thing about heavy metals is that they accumulate in the body very slowly and over time. At the same time, the body has almost no ways to free itself of them.

Normally, our body is an absolute marvel and it has adapted to many environmental conditions over the long history of mankind. Man can survive in space, we can survive in the Arctic at extreme cold temperatures as well as in the desert in extreme heat. From generation to generation, the body has been able to adapt better and better to certain environmental conditions.

On the other hand, we have not yet gotten used to heavy metals at all. This is mainly because heavy metals have been **underground** for many millennia. Only in the last few decades have large amounts of them been used for industrial production and they have thus spread rapidly.

The fundamental problem with heavy metals is that they can be stored **inside cells.** Once they have entered the cell, they disrupt the cell functions and cause it to act incorrectly. The best example of such faulty reactions are autoimmune diseases, when the immune defense is directed against the body's own tissues. Heavy metals can also damage the nerves within the cell, or they block receptors that are actually reserved for messenger substances and hormones. The damage that heavy metals can cause in the body is therefore immense.

How is the heavy metal load measured?

There is quite a large market including various providers of heavy metal tests. Unfortunately, many of these tests will give you a completely wrong result. Examples of this are heavy metal tests using blood or using hair.

A measurement by a hair sample only tells how many heavy metals are stored in the hair. In principle, the body can store heavy metals anywhere and since hair gets cut, this measurement can only provide information about the last weeks or months.

The same is true for taking a measurement from the blood. The body does not store the metals in the blood and carry them around in the body all the time. Preferentially, it stores them in some tissue. But when heavy metals are stored somewhere in tissue, then you can't get any further by measuring them in the blood.

There are all kinds of most adventurous methods for measuring heavy metal loads: From some light devices to vibration machines, everything is offered nowadays. The only thing that is made lighter for you by using such measurements is your wallet.

However, you don't have to be satisfied with such poor testing methods. A **chelation test** makes a scientifically very reliable method available and it is considered by environmental physicians to be the most reliable heavy metal test at present [14].

For the chelation test, EDTA is used in combination with DMSA or with DMSO. I will spare you the written variant of EDTA and DMSO. They are long chemical terms and looking at them this will only lead to histamine problems in the eye.

The chelation heavy metal test can be performed by a specialized doctor or alternative practitioner. As a patient, you don't have to do much at all. You only have to sit and wait for about 1.5 hours until the chelate infusion has run through. After that, a urine sample is taken and sent to a laboratory – that's it.

The following metals can be tested in a laboratory:

aluminum	mercury
arsenic	molybdenum
barium	nickel
cadmium	palladium
chrome	platinum
cobalt	silver
copper	thallium
gold	tin
lead	titanium
manganese	zinc

The chelates in the infusion act like a magnet. They circulate in the blood and attract metals. This continues until the chelates are fully saturated. The major advantage here is that the blood moves through the entire body and the stored heavy metals can be collected anywhere in the body.

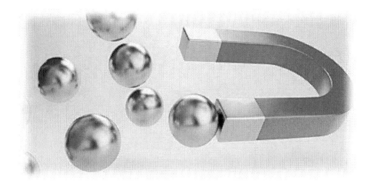

The chelates, with their bound heavy metals, are then excreted through the urine and the result can be analyzed in the laboratory. The chelation test was originally developed in the 1950s. At that time, the aim of the doctors was to rid miners of the heavy metals they had ingested underground.

What can be done to deal with heavy metals in the body?
As we have seen, testing for heavy metals is easy: The urine is collected after a chelation infusion and it is then sent to a laboratory. This then tells you how heavily your body is loaded with heavy metals. If the values are conspicuously high, then therapy should follow. For the therapy, the exact same chelation infusions are used. The only difference is that the urine is not sent to the laboratory all the time afterwards.

Before you decide on chelation therapy, it is essential to check whether your kidneys are functioning well. To do this, kidney function is measured by the value **"cystatin C."** After the chelation therapy, the heavy metals will be excreted through the urine and therefore good kidney function is very important.

However, successful heavy metal detoxification takes some patience. Over the years, many heavy metals have accumulated in your body and the chelates can only bind a certain amount of metals at a time. Therefore, you can't immediately eliminate all heavy metals with just one single chelate infusion.

Directly after the chelate infusion, it is very important to use another infusion that consists of good minerals. The chelates do not just bind the heavy metals. They also bind some good minerals, which are then excreted through the urine.

Heavy metal detoxification is very important in order to get rid of existing metals, and many histamine sufferers have already benefited enormously from this process. However, prevention is just as important as elimination, so that less heavy metals accumulate in the future.

As mentioned before, nowadays contact with heavy metals cannot be completely avoided. However, the risk can be minimized significantly by:

√ Do not wrap food in aluminum foil
√ Do not scrape around in aluminum pots and only use "soft" materials for stirring

√ Vaccinations contain aluminum - it gets directly into the blood without a protective barrier
√ Don´t use food cans (aluminum)
√ Always allow tap water to drain for some time before drinking it
√ Saltwater fish from the sea usually contains large amounts of heavy metals
√ Don´t use deodorant with aluminum

Another cause for heavy metal contamination can be an existing amalgam filling. However, you should not start on a quick fix here. There are certain cases when the removal of an amalgam filling has only triggered worse problems.

When the amalgam is drilled out, toxic mercury vapors are produced. These vapors are quickly absorbed through the oral mucosa. Therefore, it is important that an amalgam removal is only performed by a dentist who is specialized in this process.

Protective precautions when removing amalgam include protective gums for the teeth, special suction to remove the mercury vapor, removal of the amalgam in pieces (instead of drilling), and much more. If the amalgam is simply removed without further protective measures, then it may well be that a large amount of mercury enters the body.

Although the mercury exposure from amalgam fillings actually occurs in the mouth, it can affect the entire body and also trigger histamine intolerance. Mercury enters the blood through the oral mucosa and can accumulate anywhere in the body. And since heavy metals affect basic bodily functions, amalgam poisoning can then lead to a wide variety of symptoms.

I would not recommend getting an already existing amalgam filling removed as a first step. There are much better options to start treatment for histamine intolerance. However, it is important to make sure that amalgam is **not used in new fillings**. In many dental practices, amalgam is no longer even offered, but unfortunately the realization that amalgam is toxic has not yet become widespread. This is actually quite a pity, because there are much better alternatives that do not contain mercury and heavy metals.

In addition to chelation therapy, it is also possible to eliminate heavy metals using herbs. Wild garlic, coriander and chlorella algae are suitable for this purpose. However, this treatment has two decisive disadvantages compared to chelation therapy.

The herbs must first pass through the entire gastrointestinal tract. In the intestine, a certain portion of them is already lost and the heavy metal binding is mainly limited to the intestine. Therefore, detoxification using herbs can sometimes extend over a very long period of time.

In addition, the intestines of histamine sufferers are usually very agitated and sensitive already. Therefore, trying a herbal cure via the intestine would not be very advisable. Chelates, on the other hand, are administered by infusion.

This approach spares the already agitated intestine and the chelates can collect metals from any place in the body.

The second major disadvantage of using chlorella algae in particular is that it can already be heavily contaminated with heavy metals before it is even ingested. The algae are grown in water and, due to their strong attraction to heavy metals, it can be that the chlorella algae have already soaked up heavy metals if they were cultivated in polluted waters. Then you would be adding even more heavy metals to your body via the chlorella algae, and that´s the exact opposite of what you want.

Overall, I see a heavy metal test as extremely useful if you suffer from histamine intolerance. Since heavy metals accumulate slowly in the body, quite a lot of heavy metals can accumulate over the years. And at some point, there is simply too much in the body and health problems can arise as a result.

Info-Box

✓ Heavy metals can cause a lot of damage, as they are mostly stored inside cells

✓ The body usually cannot rid itself of heavy metals on its own

✓ A very reliable method to measure heavy metals in the body are chelate infusions. It´s important to get a mineral infusion right after the chelate infusion to refill good minerals

✓ Before the infusion, the function of the kidneys should be checked (via "Cystatin-C" value)

✓ Precaution is very important, therefore heavy metal exposure should be avoided in everyday life as much as possible

3.6 Up and down again: The hormones

There is a very close connection between histamine intolerance and hormones, and the female hormone "estrogen" is particularly prominent here.

The connection between hormones and histamine is impressively demonstrated during pregnancy. Throughout this time, DAO levels are increased about 500 to 1000 times [15]. A normal DAO level in a healthy person should be greater than 10 units/ml. Pregnant women can have DAO values around 5,000-10,000 units/ml. Therefore, during pregnancy, the histamine symptoms in pregnant women are usually as good as gone.

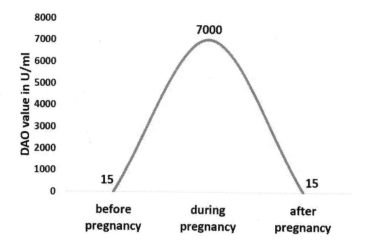

Figure 2: Example of the enormous increase in DAO level during pregnancy.

Producing so many DAO enzymes is, of course, an absolute dream state for every histamine sufferer. However, it would not be a great idea to become permanently pregnant just to get your histamine intolerance under control. That would be going a bit too far, but fortunately there are simpler solutions to histamine problems.

The hormone balance is a very sophisticated system. Not only do the individual hormones have their own spectrum of action, but they are often needed as counterparts of other hormones or messenger substances.

The best example of this is the hormone insulin, which has become quite well-known because it plays a crucial role in diabetes. Insulin ensures that the cells throughout the body are supplied with glucose, since sugar is one of the most important sources of energy for us.

In addition, insulin ensures that the blood sugar level does not rise too high after meals. When the sugar level is increased, the body activates insulin and this allows the blood sugar to be transported into the cells. Without insulin, there would be excessive amount of sugar in the blood at some point.

However, insulin can only act in one direction: If the blood glucose level is too high, then it can lower it. But what happens when the blood glucose level gets too low? Then there is not much that insulin can do here. Instead, the hormone glucagon enters the playing field.

Glucagon ensures that the liver releases glucose into the blood, thereby raising the blood sugar level again. This protects the body from dangerous hypoglycemia (low blood sugar level). For this reason, the hormone glucagon is the antagonist of the hormone insulin and they are closely connected to each other [16].

The dosage of hormones is only in the milligram or even in the microgram range. For the birth control pill, only around 0.03 milligrams of estrogen are often used. Converted into grams, that's only 0.00002 grams. This tiny amount alone has such a strong effect that a woman doesn't become pregnant. It is so little that you wouldn't even feel this tiny amount on your fingertip. This is a good way to see what a powerful effect even the smallest amounts of hormones can have on us, and how fragile and sensitive the entire hormone system is.

Since the female hormone estrogen in particular plays an important role in histamine intolerance, we will therefore take a closer look at it.

The following factors can change the estrogen balance:

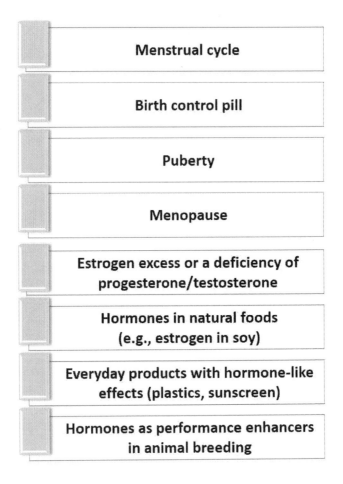

Menstrual cycle

Birth control pill

Puberty

Menopause

Estrogen excess or a deficiency of progesterone/testosterone

Hormones in natural foods (e.g., estrogen in soy)

Everyday products with hormone-like effects (plastics, sunscreen)

Hormones as performance enhancers in animal breeding

There is not much women can do about puberty, the menstrual cycle or menopause; these hormonal fluctuations are naturally predetermined. However, you have much more influence on the other factors.

Soybeans, for example, contain so-called phytoestrogens. These plant substances can have an effect that is similar to the body's own estrogen. You won't notice any effect after just consuming them once, but it will definitely have an effect if you consume soy regularly over a longer time.

On the one hand, soy is generally not recommended for anyone with histamine intolerance, because it contains histamine itself. On the other hand, the estrogen-like effect of soy ensures poorer production of DAO enzyme. Soy is a good example that even natural foods can have an influence on the hormonal system.

Besides soy, meat can also influence the hormone system. Not necessarily by nature, but more due to the conditions in animal breeding. An example from cattle breeding illustrates the dilemma: Bulls generally grow about 8-12% faster than their castrated counterparts, the steers. Therefore, the hormone loss in the steers must be compensated for in order to achieve more growth.

For this purpose, an implant with estradiol is inserted in the steer. Estradiol belongs to the group of estrogen hormones, and in ruminants, this female hormone has a restorative effect on the male animals. This artificial estrogen is, of course, then later found in the meat.

However, not only does estrogen weaken our DAO enzyme, but an elevated estrogen level additionally leads to the release of the body's own histamine. The stored histamine comes primarily from the mast cells. These are cells of the immune system that can release histamine when needed.

Mast cells are mainly located in the gastrointestinal tract, the respiratory organs, the skin, in the uterus and ovaries. Histamine problems often worsen at the onset of menstruation, during ovulation and during menopause, as estrogen levels rises during this time [17].

However, to prevent estrogen levels from constantly shooting up uncontrollably, there is a counterpart: progesterone. This is also a female hormone. It prevents an excess of estrogen from developing and, very importantly for us, progesterone inhibits the release of histamine from the mast cells. Progesterone does not stand alone, but works together with testosterone as an estrogen antagonist.

How can the hormone level be measured?
As we have seen, excess estrogen can have a negative effect on histamine intolerance. And sometimes the estrogen excess is even the fundamental cause of the development of histamine intolerance.

However, not only estrogen is important; it must always be considered in connection with some other hormones. Therefore, testing for several hormones can be useful:

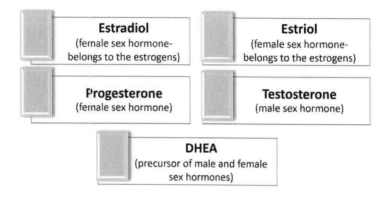

Estradiol (female sex hormone- belongs to the estrogens)	Estriol (female sex hormone- belongs to the estrogens)
Progesterone (female sex hormone)	Testosterone (male sex hormone)

DHEA
(precursor of male and female
sex hormones)

While a blood test is often useful for checking other hormones, sex hormones should be checked by a saliva test.

All the steroid hormones mentioned above are very fat-loving. This means that they bind with a fat molecule in the blood. However, this binding means that these hormones can no longer be active. Only a small proportion floats around freely in the blood and is effective.

In a blood sample, you would examine all hormones occurring in the blood. That means, examining a very large proportion of those fat-bound and deactivated molecules as well as some free hormones. This gives a total quantity of hormones, but no distinction is made between the (active) free hormones and the (inactive) bound hormones.

On the other hand, in saliva only the active hormones are naturally present. Moreover, taking a saliva sample has another advantage. Since hormones fluctuate throughout the day and they are dependent on several factors such as the menstrual cycle, multiple samples should generally be taken to create a daily profile [18].

For a blood sample, this would mean an appointment at the doctor multiple times a day. A saliva sample, on the other hand, can be taken easily at home or at work. The hormones in the saliva sample can be stored for several days at room temperature and many laboratories now offer this type of hormone testing.

However, if the following factors are present prior to saliva collection, they can falsify the measured value and should therefore be avoided:

- Smoking, brushing teeth, eating or drinking (except water)
- Bleeding gums or dental treatment shortly before measurement
- Hormone preparations (creams, pills, etc.)
- Soy products or other natural hormone stimulators
- High sports activity just before sampling

In addition to measuring hormones, it may also be useful to measure **thyroid levels.** This is because the thyroid gland also produces hormones that play an important role in your overall hormone balance.

If the thyroid values do not turn out so well, treatment using artificial hormone drugs should only be administered if it is absolutely unavoidable. Even though these drugs are often prescribed by doctors, they can do more harm than good. In this case, it is better to use natural remedies first and an improvement in lifestyle habits can sometimes work wonders.

How can the hormone balance be brought back into equilibrium?

If you suspect that histamine intolerance has arisen due to an imbalance in hormone levels, then consulting an expert in this field is worthwhile.

The first step is always to take a saliva measurement to check scientifically whether there is any estrogen dominance at all. Taking further action is only reasonable if the saliva measurement results are conspicuous. A normal functioning hormone balance should never be interfered with! If you want to get your hormonal balance back, then always only do this in a gentle and natural way first.

Often the estrogen level decreases with age. This would actually be ideal for histamine intolerance, because estrogen releases the histamine stored in the body and also blocks the DAO enzyme. But unfortunately, the progesterone level also decreases with age, and much faster than the estrogen level.

This is why estrogen dominance develops with increasing age, especially in women. The ratio of estrogen and its counterparts becomes unbalanced and there is either too much estrogen or too little of the opposite hormones.

Another hint, that the hormonal balance plays a very important role is shown by the fact that histamine intolerance affects around 75% women, mostly at the age of 35 years or older [19].

113

To counteract the estrogen surplus somewhat, there are some foods that restore the hormone balance quite naturally. These include cauliflower, broccoli and especially kale. These foods are rich in indole-3-carbinol and regulate hormone balance.

Other natural hormone stabilizers are pomegranate, fennel, yams, monk's pepper, coconut oil, ghee, quinoa and brown rice. Organic foods are preferable, because they contain very little to no pesticides, and pesticides can also affect hormone balance. Even if the foods mentioned are low in histamine, you should check slowly to see if you can tolerate them.

Quite a lot can be done by eating a hormone-balancing diet. However, the whole process really gets moving when you optimize your lifestyle habits. The following factors have a negative effect on hormone balance and should therefore be avoided:

- Vitamin D deficiency
- Stimulants such as nicotine or caffeine
- Too little movement
- Too much stress
- Certain medicines
- Environmental pollutants
- Heavy metal contamination
- Foods that contain hormones themselves (for example, meat or soy products)
- Ready-made meals
- Pesticides (for example, in fruits and vegetables)
- Permanent lack of sleep

- Nutrient deficiencies (vitamins, minerals and a lack of omega 3 fatty acids)
- Hormones in tap water (use water filter)

Although it is often tedious to constantly discipline ourselves, lifestyle habits are hugely important to our health, and this includes diet as well as everyday lifestyle.

If this method does not help, natural hormones can also be used in consultation with an experienced therapist. They can be obtained from the yam root or other natural sources. But as already mentioned, you should approach the whole matter of hormones very carefully.

Info-Box

✓ During pregnancy, DAO level increases by about 500 to 1000 times

✓ The estrogen level plays an important role in histamine intolerance: It can release the body's own histamine and also block the DAO enzyme

✓ To check hormones, a saliva test is much more reliable than a blood test

✓ Hormone balance can be improved, by eating certain foods, reducing stress and exercising regularly

3.7   Medications and alcohol

We have already seen, that the DAO enzyme can come under fire from many sides. For example, unbalanced intestinal flora, a lack of nutrients or heavy metal toxicity can be responsible for this. But there are a few more factors that can put a strain on your DAO and thus trigger or aggravate histamine intolerance. Two of these critical factors are alcohol as well as medications.

Medications

Medications include not only pills and tablets, but also creams or effervescent tablets. Although most medications themselves usually do not contain histamine at all, they can still release histamine stored in the body or block our famous DAO enzyme.

For example, anti-inflammatory painkillers containing the substances mefenamic acid or diclofenac are critical, because these substances release a lot of histamine in the body.

When a lot of histamine is released by a medication, then allergy-like symptoms often appear, such as skin rashes. With these symptoms, many doctors usually think of a type I allergy. A typical characteristic for an allergy (in contrast to histamine intolerance) is, that the **immune system becomes active**. In this case, it is possible to measure if your symptoms come from an allergy by testing IgE-antibodies in the blood and with an additional skin test.

When symptoms come from a histamine reaction only, then the allergy test in the blood and on the skin will be negative. Therefore, allergy-like symptoms can occur after taking a medication, and they can be triggered by histamine. It then appears like an allergy, but it isn´t one. However, it is also possible for histamine sufferers to have a true allergy and histamine intolerance at the same time.

When a drug releases the body´s own histamine, then the symptoms are usually felt after a short time. In addition to histamine-releasing drugs, there are also drugs that block DAO enzyme. These include, for example, expectorant and analgesic drugs containing the substances acetylcysteine or metamizole. Here, the intolerance reaction does not show up immediately, but only after the next meal.

The reason for the time delay is that these drugs inhibit DAO enzyme activity. If a subsequent meal then contains a lot of histamine, the DAO enzymes are not available to completely break down the histamine from the food. The whole process is quite insidious, because the symptoms are delayed and they are usually not associated with taking the medication.

There are so many medications on the market nowadays that it is difficult to keep track of which medications are tolerated by histamine sufferers and which are not. Here too, it is crucial to know in the first place that not only food but also medications can lead to a histamine reaction.

Knowing this may suddenly explain ominous, unexplained reactions to medications or ointments. And when you know that you get histamine symptoms from certain medications, then you can try to get an alternative medication.

Contrast agents and anesthetics

Not only medications can be critical in histamine intolerance, but also anesthetics before a surgery as well as contrast media for X-ray, computed tomography (CT) and magnetic resonance imaging (MRI) examinations.

During an examination by X-ray, CT or MRI, a **contrast medium** is almost always administered. This makes it much easier to distinguish between organs, and it also helps to identify inflammations or tumors with a good blood supply [20].

However, as helpful as the contrast media are during the examination, they can cause various reactions in histamine sufferers. Particularly in X-rays, it is known that all contrast media used to date lead to a strong histamine release.

Administration of the contrast agent causes the histamine level in the body to rise sharply. While this may be noticeable in a healthy person by a feeling of warmth during the examination, histamine sufferers have to contend with much stronger reactions. Therefore, it is important that you discuss your histamine intolerance with the doctor or radiologist in advance.

It is by now known that there are typical high-risk patients for X-ray, CT or MRI examinations – such as patients with weak kidneys or allergy sufferers. However, the fact that someone with histamine intolerance can also develop health problems from contrast media is unfortunately hardly known.

However, a histamine reaction can be counteracted well by administering an H1 and H2 antihistamine before the examination. The body still releases the same amount of histamine, but the antihistamine blocks the histamine receptors and thus the strong histamine reactions do not occur.

Since the contrast media are excreted via the kidneys, it is recommended that you drink plenty of fluids after the examination. The faster the contrast media are out of the body again, the better.

Histamine intolerance should therefore be discussed with the physician or anesthesiologist at an early stage before **surgery**, because anesthetics can also lead to histamine release.

In Appendix 1 you will find an overview of anesthetics, narcotics and X-ray contrast media provided from Charité Berlin University Hospital. This overview was created for mastocytosis patients. However, the guidelines also apply to histamine sufferers, since increased histamine levels cause problems in both groups.

Alcohol

Although alcohol contains significantly less histamine than fish or long-aged cheese, it is still a major trigger for histamine intolerance.

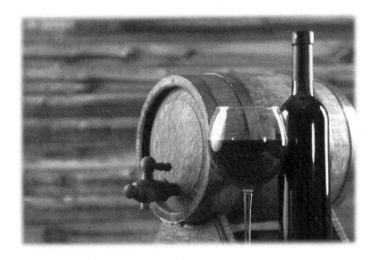

While most foods or beverages simply contain too much histamine, alcohol has four negative effects:

1. Alcohol increases the permeability of the intestinal mucosa. This attacks the natural protective barrier of the intestine
2. Alcohol inhibits the activity of DAO enzyme
3. It releases histamine stored in the body (histamine liberator)

4. Alcohol contains biogenic amines that compete with histamine degradation and are degraded prior to histamine

Well, that's pretty bad news for anyone who likes a drink. But with alcohol too "the dose makes the poison," and a glass of alcohol now and then will not be a fundamental cause of histamine intolerance. However, if you drink larger quantities every day, then the intestinal flora and mucous membrane are severely affected. In the long run, this can increase histamine intolerance and damage the intestine.

Ideally, in case of histamine intolerance should you abstain completely from alcohol. However, everyday life is usually somewhat different and there are also many people who simply like to drink a glass for pleasure.

The histamine content in alcoholic beverages can vary greatly. During the process of ripening, the histamine content also increases. A certain amount of histamine in a drink is already determined at harvest. For example, the more microorganism grapes and their stems contain at harvest, the higher the proportion of biogenic amines in the beverage later on.

Wine and sparkling wine: Red wine in particular usually contains a high amount of histamine. In contrast, white wine or sparkling wine contain comparatively less histamine. In red wine, lactic acid bacteria are often used during fermentation, so that the acid in the wine is broken down.

Due to this acid degradation, red wines contain significantly more histamine.

However, the sulfite in white wine and sparkling wine can also cause problems, because it releases the body's own histamine. Generally, storage in wooden barrels or barriques leads to a significantly higher histamine content in the wine. Fresh grape must, on the other hand, is low in histamine.

So, when buying wine, the following applies: Young wines with a short fermentation process should be preferred and the wine should not be stored for a long time. The longer you store wine (or anything else), the more time there is for histamine to build up in it. By contrast, white wine without biological acid degradation is significantly easier to tolerate than red wine. The more the acid in the wine has been degraded, the higher the histamine content.

Nowadays, there are many suppliers of wine on the Internet who offer wine especially made for histamine sufferers. These wines are tested for their histamine content and thus already jump the first hurdle: They themselves contain almost no histamine.

Even though a histamine-free wine sounds very tempting, you should still keep in mind that these wines can still cause problems. They might not contain histamine, but they can contain **biogenic amines,** which then can make the breakdown of histamine from food more difficult later on.

In addition, the **alcohol** in wine reduces DAO enzyme activity and it can also release the histamine stored in the body. A "histamine-free" wine is therefore by no means a free pass. However, in smaller quantities, it can be significantly more digestible than commercial wine.

Beer: The histamine content of beer also varies between types and different manufacturers. The main differences are between top-fermented and bottom-fermented beer.

Top-fermented beer usually contains significantly more histamine than bottom-fermented beer. The term top-fermented comes from the fact that during fermentation the yeast floats on top of the brew, and then only needs to be skimmed off. Here, the yeast works at temperatures about 15-20° C.

Bottom-fermented beer, on the other hand, contains significantly less histamine. Here, the yeast works at temperatures around 4-9°C and it then settles at the bottom of the vat.

Spirits: Of all spirits, the clear ones are the most tolerable. In contrast, liqueurs with a high sugar content, as well as barrel-aged spirits like whiskey and cognac, have a significantly higher histamine content. [6].

In histamine intolerance, alcohol is generally less well tolerated when it is

- drunk warm
- carbonated
- drunk quickly
- drunk on an empty stomach
- contains sugar
- consumed in large quantities
- contains incompatible fruit extracts or preservatives
- contains sulfites
- colored with artificial dyes

Basically, you should be aware that alcohol is generally not very beneficial in case of histamine intolerance. And the more you drink, the more damage it can do. As so often, the amount makes the poison.

However, there is also good news for those who have drinks very regularly, because the excessive alcohol consumption could be the main trigger for histamine intolerance. This means, by reducing or quitting your drinking, the histamine intolerance can improve significantly.

Info-Box

- ✓ Drugs can release the body's own histamine (histamine releasers) or inhibit the activity of the DAO enzyme
- ✓ Contrast media used in X-ray, CT or MRI examination almost all release histamine. Here, the administration of an H1 and H2 antihistamine can help
- ✓ Anesthetics before surgery can also release histamine - talk to the doctor or anesthesiologist in advance
- ✓ Alcohol is bad for histamine intolerance in several ways: It contains histamine, blocks the DAO enzyme, it contains biogenic amines that inhibit histamine breakdown and it releases body's own histamine

3.8 Other treatment options

So far, we have already looked at several important causes of histamine intolerance. But there can be several other triggers for histamine intolerance as well. If you are completely new to the topic of histamine intolerance, I would recommend that you first take the measures described in the previous chapters. These are the main ones and I would suggest to tackle them first.

The measures include a stool sample to analyze the condition of the intestine, tests for other foods you can't tolerate (fructose, lactose and gluten), and measurement of DAO enzyme as well as co-factors such as copper, zinc and vitamin B6 in whole blood.

When you have taken these measures, you can build up a good basis and have enough to do for the time being. And for many patients, these measures have also led to the fastest results in the past. A good diagnosis is very important and therefore it is crucial to use reliable scientific tests.

For a good diagnosis, you should avoid tests like light ray measurement, bioresonance, kinesiology or similar methods. This is not to say that bioresonance or kinesiology are generally bad. But for measuring intestinal flora, heavy metals, vitamins in the body and much more, there are better options nowadays. Fortunately, we live in an age of science and we should take advantage of this fact.

In science, certain basic principles and quality criteria prevail. These include objectivity, validity and reliability. The fact that a test must be reliable is absolutely crucial for patients. When you get a result, you really need to trust it.

Also, you pay money for a test and above all, you or your therapist will base the further procedures on the test result. A diagnosis is the foundation for the subsequent treatments. If the testing method is wrong and delivers false results, then the treatment just can´t work, because it is based on false assumptions. Therefore, we will take a short excursion into science and look at what are these criteria for a good test.

Objectivity means that the measurement results are completely independent of the person making the measurement. If another researcher does the same experiment, he should come to exactly the same result. Thus, no one can fudge the results. For example, if you send a blood sample to two different laboratories to have your vitamin D level determined and both laboratories use the exact same method, then they should come to the exact same result.

Validity means that the measurement follows a logical concept. You can't measure the length of your little finger and then make a statement about the pH value of your intestine. There is no connection between the finger and the pH value in the intestine. At least, none is known to me. However, if you measure the pH value by means of a stool sample instead of the length of the little finger, then you can already make much more precise statements about the pH value of the intestine.

Another example of a measurement with no validity would be a hair analysis to test for heavy metals. In this kind of test, a few hairs from the head are tested for various heavy metals. It is even possible to determine the amount of heavy metals from hair very accurately in a laboratory.

However, heavy metals can be stored anywhere in the body. Therefore, the heavy metal content in hair says nothing about the heavy metals elsewhere in the body. And besides, you can only see the part that has been stored in the hair. In addition, hair is cut regularly and a hair analysis only lets you see the amount of heavy metals that were stored within the last months. Therefore, hair analysis is not a suitable, scientific method to measure the heavy metal load in the body. The procedure itself is fine, but it is the wrong place of measurement and in the end, it will give you false results.

And finally, there is also **reliability**. This means that the same result is obtained when the measurement is repeated in exactly the same way. Reliability therefore means how accurate and reliable the measurement is.

Reliability is very important for lab tests. During my internship at Mercedes Benz in the U.S., we had a transport company called "Reliable.". The reliability of a transport company is very important in that kind of business and my boss used to make this joke "Is Reliable reliable?" and that´s how I remember how important reliability is.

But why am I telling you so much about science and accurate test results on the subject of histamine intolerance? Unfortunately, there are many dubious profiteers who make a lot of money performing literally hair-raising tests. As a consequence, the patients get wrong results and also lose a lot of money.

You might hope that there are only a few rip-offs in this industry. But right off the bat, I can think of more than six test procedures or companies that I myself fell for and unfortunately, I burned away a lot of money with them.

There were companies who claimed to cure intolerances with just a spit test or another institute that claimed to measure the intolerance of 300 foods at once, just using a little blood. At another place, a pendulum was used to check my blood and I was told that I had certain parasites and heavy metals in my body. This is all very scary and I wouldn´t believe it, if I had not experienced it myself!

In addition, there are all the stories that many readers have sent me already. Bad tests for histamine intolerance and irritable bowel syndrome are therefore not at all a rarity, but rather the normal case.

You pay for the test and therefore, you have the right to get a good and reliable test result. But what is even worse than losing the money: Your further treatment will be based on this false test result.

Let's say you are told, as the result of an ominous IgG antibody measurement, that you do not have histamine intolerance at all. According to this test, it says that instead from histamine you suffer from lactose intolerance. You now change your entire diet to lactose-free, use your limited free time to research about lactose intolerance and you tell your friends that you can't eat milk products anymore.

However, you continue to eat products containing histamine, because the test for histamine was supposedly negative. And after a couple weeks, you wonder why your health still hasn't improved at all. You might even think that you haven't worked hard enough or you cheated too often in your diet. But the answer as to why nothing has improved, is quite simple – a completely wrong test was to blame.

If, on the other hand, you had done a breath test for lactose intolerance, then you would have known very well if you can tolerate products containing lactose. And if you additionally do a histamine omission diet for three weeks and determine your DAO blood level, then you also know quite precisely whether you have histamine intolerance. Once you have done a good testing process, then you can make adjustments to everything else – from diet, supplements up to therapy. And the good thing is, that you only have to do these tests once.

Below I have listed the best and most reliable testing options currently available for each food intolerance:

Intolerance	Currently best testing option
Histamine intolerance	- Elimination diet (avoid histamine) for about 3 weeks - Measure DAO value and total histamine level in blood
Lactose intolerance	- Hydrogen breath test for lactose
Fructose intolerance	- Hydrogen breath test for fructose

Gluten intolerance (celiac disease)	- Elimination diet (omit gluten) for about 3 weeks
	- Blood test for:
	  –> Transglutaminase-IgA
	  –> Endomysium-IgA
	  –> Total-IgA

Table 3: How to find out if you suffer from food intolerance

Besides the most common causes for histamine intolerance already mentioned, there are a few more possible causes that can trigger histamine intolerance as well.

HPU

And here comes the next technical term! Fortunately, the abbreviation "HPU" has become the established term, because the long form "hemopyrrollactamuria" is definitely a tongue twister.

The disease HPU is a metabolic disorder that, if left untreated, often leads to digestive and histamine problems. Although there are many different metabolic disorders, such as diabetes, hyperthyroidism or gout, HPU in particular is closely associated with the development of histamine intolerance.

A metabolic disease – that somehow doesn't sound good. But HPU is not that bad and testing for HPU does not hurt at all. Once detected, HPU can be managed very well. As it is the case so often, it is crucial to detect HPU at all. In most cases, HPU is inherited, but it can sometimes develop over the course of life and women are affected 10 times more often than men.

But what exactly is HPU? When we breathe in, we absorb oxygen through the lungs. The oxygen from the lungs must then be distributed throughout the body. To do this, the oxygen binds to the red blood cells, the hemoglobin.

Hemoglobin is like a packhorse and transports oxygen everywhere in the body. And as the name suggests, hemoglobin is made up from heme (an iron complex) and globin (a protein compound). Both the heme and the globin can be produced by the body itself.

In HPU disease, there is a disturbance in the production of this heme. As a result of this disorder, normal, "good" heme is produced, but at the same time a certain amount of "false" heme is also produced. The body naturally wants to get rid of this "false" heme, but it cannot do this on its own. Therefore, it has to bind the false heme to vitamin B6, zinc and partly to manganese, so that it can excrete the heme via the urine.

Wait a minute: Vitamin B6, zinc and manganese... Weren't these exactly the substances that are so important for the formation of DAO enzyme? This means, that due to HPU metabolic disease, the body consumes exactly those vitamins and minerals that we need so urgently for the activation of DAO enzyme.

With HPU metabolic disease, a certain amount of the "false" heme is formed every day. Therefore, the body has to take something from its vital substance balance every day in order to dispose the false heme. And in the process, it consumes a particularly large amount of vitamin B6, zinc and manganese.

As a result, important vital substances that are actually needed for other processes are used up over time. In everyday life, the body is simultaneously burdened with other pollutants from the environment in addition to the "false" heme.

However, due to HPU, the body is significantly less able to dispose of these pollutants, since it has already used the necessary nutrients to dispose of the "false" heme. Thus, two problem areas arise at the same time due to HPU: A lack of nutrients (vitamin B6, zinc and manganese) as well as a limited detoxification capacity.

How do you check for HPU?
Checking for HPU is quite simple and painless by testing 24-hour urine. To do this, you simply collect your urine over 24 hours and then send a small sample of it to the laboratory.

The excretion of HPU complexes can vary greatly throughout the day. However, the 24-hour test is not affected by this, because by collecting the urine over 24 hours, fluctuations throughout the day are well balanced out and a reliable test result is obtained.

Sometimes the so-called KPU test is used to check for HPU disease. The KPU test measures the cryptopyrroluria complexes. However, the KPU test can be distorted by certain foods, medications or stress.

The HPU test, on the other hand, measures a very specific chemical compound that is only formed during the formation of the "false" heme. Unfortunately, the KPU test is still quite often used to measure for HPU disease, maybe because both names sound similar. But only the HPU test is the more reliable one here.

It should be noted that about two weeks before having a HPU test, no food supplements such as B vitamins or zinc should be taken, because these can falsify the test result. For testing I can recommend the KEAC laboratory in the Netherlands, which offers the HPU test[1].

When there is no option of finding a laboratory to test for HPU, then there is another way that can give an indication of HPU disease. When someone has HPU, their body will have a significantly higher consumption of vitamin B6, zinc and manganese. Therefore, when you measure these nutrients in whole blood, their values would be noticeably low.

What can be done about HPU?
If the test has shown that HPU metabolic disorder is present, then the empty nutrient depots must be replenished. It is particularly important to replenish vitamin B6, zinc and manganese.

This helps the body to get out of its energy-sapping deficiency state. Because it is so important, I must point out again at this point: When taking vitamin B6, it is essential to ensure that the **active vitamin B6 (P-5-P)** is taken.

---

[1]http://www.keac.nl

Since someone with HPU usually lacks several nutrients, it is recommended that a supplement containing all B vitamins is taken for a certain period of time.

At first glance, taking nutritional supplements does not seem like a spectacular treatment concept for HPU. But in case of HPU metabolic disorder, a deficiency of certain nutrients is precisely the key of why certain processes are out of whack.

And this is precisely where this treatment comes in. Of course, it would be ideal to eliminate the cause directly, but in most cases the cause of HPU is genetic and there is not much that can be done about it.

However, for anyone with HPU, there is much more that can be done than just taking nutritional supplements. Mostly, the detoxification capacity is limited. Therefore, you should pay special attention to the foods you eat. They should be as natural as possible and above all without any toxins, since additional toxins can have a strong effect particularly on HPU sufferers.

Stress
Stress can be another reason for histamine intolerance. This includes psychological stress, such as deadline pressure, worries and fears. But there is also physical stress. The body is always under stress when it has to deal with an illness or certain environmental influences.

Our intestine is permeated with millions of nerve cells. After the brain, the intestine is the organ with the most nerve cells and that is why it is often called the "second brain." When the nerve cells in the intestine are activated by stress, they can release the stored histamine from the mast cells.

However, this amount of histamine is significantly lower than the amount consumed through food. That's why you shouldn't let your doctor tell you that your histamine symptoms are only caused by stress. A typical phrase, which many people with digestive problems have heard already is, that "Your complaints are only psychosomatic." With this advice comes usually a recommendation to go to a psychiatrist.

Those who really suffer from very severe stress should urgently do something about it. Especially the heart, but other organs as well will be very grateful for any reduction of stress, because excessive stress can do a lot of harm in the long run.

However, it is not at all possible in everyday life to be completely without anxiety, stress or anger for even a single week. It is part of life, and the body has naturally learned to cope with it. It is not decisive if we have stress, but it is much more important that we don't permanently exceed our personal limit.

If you were told that your histamine problems are only psychosomatic, then you do not need to bury your head in the sand. In the previous chapters we have seen that you can do a lot on the physical level.

That stress impacts the stomach and intestine is definitely true. But I would never blame permanent, severe digestive problems solely on the psyche. In most cases, there is much more on the physical level behind these problems. If stress really is the main cause of histamine disorder, then the symptoms should improve significantly during stress-free times, for example after a relaxing vacation.

Or conversely, the symptoms should worsen much more in very stressful, tense phases. Stress and nervous strain can theoretically be a cause of histamine intolerance, but in most cases, there are mostly also physical causes behind it.

However, there is one way in which severe stress can actually lead to histamine problems. This does not happen directly through histamine release, but through the development of a leaky gut syndrome.

The body has learned that it needs to get energy very quickly in stressful situations, such as escaping or fighting. In these moments, it expands the distance between the cells of the intestinal mucosa in order to immediately get the energy from the food that has not yet been completely digested.

The fact that the body does something like this in an emergency situation is very good and right, because it helps us to survive. But what happens when the body feels that it is on the run every day?

In this situation, a leaky gut syndrome develops again and again. The expanded distance between the cells in the intestine will lead to an inflammation and certain substances can slip through the intestinal wall. The defense reaction against these hostile substances in turn leads to the release of histamine. And due to the leaky gut, the intestine is battered and it can therefore produce significantly less of our popular DAO enzyme.

Our intestine is a very central organ in many areas. And it is symbolic that it is located very centrally in the middle of the body. However, there is not only a close connection between the intestine and the skin, but also between the intestine and the brain. This connection is called the gut-brain axis.

Not only does the intestine itself have millions of nerve cells. But also, via the gut-brain axis, psychological problems or stress can affect the intestine.

However, this is not just a one-way street into one direction; the brain and intestine can influence each other. Stress and worries can affect the intestine, but in the same way, an impaired intestine can cause various mental problems such as lack of concentration, listlessness, depression or mood swings.

Therefore, stress can affect the intestine and influence digestion. But if you are not suffering from extreme permanent stress or traumatic experiences, then you should look for the cause of your histamine intolerance much more on the physical level.

Skin

Many histamine sufferers know the connection between histamine and the skin only too well: After eating certain foods, the skin turns red or it starts itching in various places.

There are mast cells in the skin and they store the body's own histamine. We have already seen this at the beginning, about how contact with a stinging nettle leads to a histamine reaction on the skin.

In the connection of skin and histamine, there are two ways in which they influence each other. If we take in too much histamine through certain foods, then this histamine excess can show itself directly through a reaction on the skin.

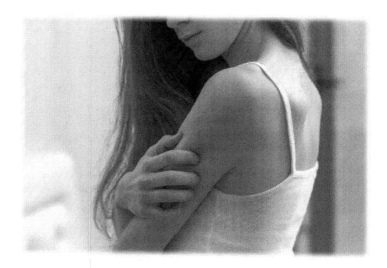

And there is also the opposite way: When the skin is irritated, it releases histamine and this creates an excess of histamine in the body. This overdose of histamine can then in turn lead to further digestive problems.

For histamine sufferers, it is important to know about this skin-and-histamine connection, because it also has an impact on everyday life. Not only food, but everything that comes into contact with the skin can lead to a histamine release and thus can lead to symptoms. This includes ointments, shower gels, tinctures or creams.

Therefore, if you have persistent histamine problems, you should not only pay attention to what you eat. It is also possible that histamine is released every day through skin contact with certain substances. And this in turn can lead to digestive problems, even though no redness or allergic reaction is visible on the skin.

Allergies

Histamine intolerance itself is not in an allergy. The most important characteristic of an allergy is that the **immune system** becomes active. This is not the case with histamine intolerance, because the immune system does not react to histamine and therefore histamine intolerance is not an allergy. However, since histamine intolerance symptoms and complaints are very similar to a real allergy, it is often referred to as a pseudo allergy.

In the case of an allergy to pollen or cat dander, the immune system has at some point mistakenly classified certain substances as an "enemy." And with every further contact, the immune system recognizes this enemy again and fights it. This fight is then also accompanied by a high output of histamine.

Therefore, it is possible that you are suffering from typical histamine problems, although there is actually enough of the good DAO enzyme available. The trigger for these histamine problems can be the allergy instead of the histamine intolerance. On contact with the allergy substances, a lot of histamine is released in the body each time and the histamine from the allergy is added additionally on top of the histamine that is already contained in food.

For this reason, the total histamine value in the blood should always be determined in addition to the DAO value. If this value is significantly above the normal value, then there is clearly too much histamine in the body. If the total amount of histamine in the body is constantly too high, then even a healthy person can no longer properly break down these excessive amounts and subsequently suffers from the typical histamine symptoms.

However, the total histamine value should be checked at least twice, because it fluctuates quite strongly on a daily basis. If you have cheese and red wine at dinner the day before, then the histamine value is naturally going to be significantly higher than if you have only rice and fresh vegetables the evening before.

If it turns out that the total histamine value is very high, then it may be that an allergy is behind it. This could be to animal dander, molds or pollen. If at the same time there is enough of the DAO enzyme present, then you probably don´t even suffer from a "real" histamine intolerance, but rather the allergy causes a huge histamine overdose in the body, which even healthy people can´t handle.

To further clarify whether there is an allergy behind your symptoms, you can do an **allergy test** for various triggers. These tests are usually offered by a dermatologist or allergist. And of course, you should keep an eye on unspecific allergy symptoms, such as a stuffy nose or certain reactions when animals are around.

3.9   Summary

We have now seen that there are many ways to get rid of your histamine intolerance. Every person is unique and everyone also has a very individual health and life story behind them. That is why there are so many different reasons for the cause of histamine intolerance.

Unfortunately, it is not so easy to keep an overview of all the possibilities and what is the best way to start?

In the following, you will find an overview of measures that I consider important and useful. The list is arranged so that the most important things are at the top, which should ideally be tested first.

Diagnose	How to test for it?
Test for histamine intolerance	- Elimination diet (avoid histamine-rich food for two to three weeks) - Measure DAO-value and total histamine value (both in blood)
Check for further food-intolerances	- Especially lactose (hydrogen breath test), fructose (hydrogen breath test) und gluten (blood test)
Disturbed intestinal flora	-Stool sample with all values mentioned before (like zonulin, alpha-1 antitrypsin, gut bacteria...) - Check function of pancreas as well with this stool sample (by "Pancreatic elastase value")
Vitamin and mineral analysis	- Check especially for copper, vitamin B6 and zinc - Try to measure as many values as possible (B vitamins, different minerals, etc.) - Vitamins and minerals have to be measured in whole blood (not in serum)
Heavy metals	- Check function of kidneys first (cystantin-c value) - Chelate-Test with EDTA and DMSA/DMSO (per infusion)
Allergy	- Get an allergy test done by a dermatologist (check for reactions to animals, house dust and pollen)
Medications	- Check which medications you are currently taking (keep in mind that drugs can release histamine and block the efficacy of DAO enzyme)
HPU metabolic disease	- HPU-test in 24h-urin - Use KPU-test only as a second option, if you can't find a laboratory that offers HPU-tests
Alcohol	- Alcohol can contain histamine, release stored histamine (histamine liberator) and block the DAO enzyme - It is essential to stop or severely limit alcohol consumption
Hormones	- Have the following hormones tested: estradiol, estriol, progesterone, testosterone and DHEA - Measure via saliva test, not in blood - Stop active hormone supply (like pill or IUD)
Stress	- Too much permanent stress can cause a release of the body's own histamine - Check if symptoms get significantly better in calm times or on vacation
HNMT enzyme	- There are no reliable test methods yet - Keep in mind, that drugs can block the power of HNMT

4 Tips and ideas for everyday life

4.1   Daily lifestyle

Movement

Getting enough exercise is very important for good digestion. But in the case of histamine intolerance, too intense exercise or high-performance sports can do more harm than good. Intense sports cause the body to release histamine, which happens even in healthy people. But if there are too few DAO enzymes, the excess histamine from sports activity is broken down too slowly and the typical histamine symptoms appear.

On the other hand, exercise is very important because it boosts many processes in the body – from metabolism to blood circulation. Especially nowadays, we spend far too much time sitting. That's why frequent exercise is very good and important, but it should be moderate and not too strenuous, because otherwise the positive benefit tips into the opposite.

Fasting

In principle, mankind had always experienced periods of hunger. If hunting was not successful or the weather hardly allowed anything to grow, then people had to starve. Supermarkets did not exist and there were no refrigerators for longer storage of the food. Only in the last 50 to 60 years has this situation been overcome and we have a constant, excessive supply of food and calories. Of course, the body always has an appetite, especially for sugar and fats.

After all, dating back to the Stone Age, our body doesn't know when there will be food the next time, and it naturally wants to store as many calories as possible to be prepared for hunger periods. Who knows when there will be something to eat again. The terms ice cream parlor, supermarket or restaurant are completely unknow to the body.

Particularly when you have a damaged intestine, it can therefore be useful to **skip a meal**. This might feel unusual in the beginning, but it is a completely natural thing for the body. Only by taking a break from eating can the intestine concentrate on **repairing and healing**.

Here as well, just try it out and see if it makes you feel better. The extreme form of this is therapeutic fasting is to go without food for several days. That is clearly more strenuous and requires also a huge portion of perseverance. But many people swear by the healing effect of fasting.

Antibiotics and preservatives
Nowadays, it is commonly known that antibiotics can take the bacterial equilibrium in the intestine out of balance. That's why there are many histamine sufferers whose dilemma only got going after taking antibiotics.

But why exactly are antibiotics so critical and how can they lead to histamine intolerance? DAO enzyme is the main requirement for the breakdown of histamine and more than 90% of this enzyme is produced in the intestine [2]. However, if the intestine has been severely affected by an antibiotic, then the production of DAO no longer runs smoothly. The consequence is a lack of DAO and therefore, histamine can no longer be broken down properly – a vicious circle.

However, antibiotics are not generally bad and there are many cases when antibiotics have saved lives. Here as well, the dose makes the poison. If antibiotics are really only used in an emergency and with care, the benefits clearly outweigh the disadvantages. And when antibiotics were taken, then a course of treatment with probiotics (products with good bacteria for the intestine) should follow directly.

Preservatives also have an effect similar to antibiotics. Preservatives are used to ensure that food products have a long shelf life. Accordingly, they are often found in convenience foods or generally in all foods that are supposed to be stored for a long time. Of course, preservatives have certain advantages, for example they last much longer and no refrigeration is necessary.

However, preservatives are anything but good for us. When they enter our intestine, they do exactly what they were created for: They kill bacteria. And this leads to the destruction of good bacteria and attacks the intestinal mucosa.

Preservatives are often found in ready-made meals and that's why fresh ingredients should be used as often as possible. Preservatives are identified on the packaging whether by their full name or as an abbreviation by the numbers E-200 to E-299.

Adequate fluid intake

You might wonder why is it recommended so often that people should drink enough water or tea? This advice must be included in any health guide, so there seems to be something to it.

First of all, the need for fluids is mainly due to the fact that humans consist of more than 70% water. Every cell, every organ needs water to be able to function at all. Even if the body wants to get rid of waste products, it has to dilute them with water in order to eliminate them. This elimination process even takes place in the field of histamine.

Histamine inside a cell is made biologically inactive by the HNMT enzyme and it is then transported to the liver. There it is converted into "N-methylimidaol-4-yl acetic acid" (of course, everyone knows this one). Subsequently, it is transported to the kidneys and then excreted into the urine. The breakdown of histamine in the body therefore leads to waste products that have to be disposed through the urine.

However, if you drink too little, then these waste products cannot be excreted properly. This is like your garbage disposal only taking half of the garbage with it. Therefore, sufficient liquid intake every day is very important, for healthy people and even more for someone with histamine intolerance.

4.2   Emergency medicine – When things get bad again

The long-term goal is to find the cause of histamine intolerance and treat it successfully. However, this requires some testing and, above all, it takes time. Before you have figured out which foods you can handle well and which you can´t, it can happen quite often that your symptoms become very severe sometimes and that they restrict your everyday life a lot. To get over this on the short run, there is certain SOS medicines that are very useful for acute phases.

Products that contain DAO enzymes: This medication should be taken around 15 minutes before a histamine-rich meal. It contains a protein extract from pig kidney or of plant origin and it is rich in DAO enzymes. This additional DAO helps to break down histamine better.

However, you should be careful. This medication should not be taken for a long time! Some people with histamine intolerance who have taken it for a longer time report, that the effect wears off quite quickly. And if you take it for a longer time, it can even aggravate your symptoms, because the intestine now thinks that it constantly has enough DAO, it gets lazy and produces much less of it.

Healing clay and zeolite: Both remedies can help with detoxification and bind histamine in the intestine.

Antihistamines: These are the classic histamine emergency medications. For histamine to exert its effect at all, it must bind to a histamine receptor in the body. There are four types: H1 to H4 receptors.

When you take an antihistamine, it attaches to these receptor sites, but without triggering an effect. As a result, the receptor is occupied and histamine can no longer dock there. The effect is similar to a parking space that is already occupied by the antihistamine. Most antihistamines are available in pharmacies.

The antihistamines on the market nowadays are focused on blocking the H1 as well as the H2 receptor. The H1 receptor is mainly responsible for dilated blood vessels, itchy or red skin, the day-night rhythm and the contraction of smooth muscles in the intestine (diarrhea). The H2 receptor, on the other hand, induces higher gastric juice production, accelerated heart rate and increased mucus production in the respiratory tract.

Okoubaka: "Okoubaka aubrevillei" is a jungle tree of the sandalwood family and grows in West Africa. To obtain the medicine, the bark is first dried and then processed into powder. Long before okoubaka became known to us, the tribes and healers in West Africa used it.

This remedy is available in the form of globules or drops. It acts primarily in the gastrointestinal tract and is generally helpful for gastrointestinal problems. It also has a detoxifying effect and a stimulating effect on the immune system.

As already mentioned, all these SOS remedies mentioned are intended only for emergencies. They only help against the symptoms, which is important in acute situations. But in the long term, the focus should definitely be on finding the cause and thus **curing** the disease and not just suppressing the symptoms.

4.3   Making your piggy bank happy: Financial tips & ideas

Theoretically, you could start with the treatment right away... But only theoretically, because there is still a big catch in the whole thing – and that is the dear money. Since most of these treatments costs are not covered by health insurances, you always have to think about whether you can afford a treatment or not.

However, even though these treatments are usually not billable through your health insurance, there are some ways to recoup a large portion of the cost.

Since the majority of doctors unfortunately do not offer any treatment at all for histamine intolerance, most of the patients go to an alternative practitioner. And there can be suitable supplementary insurances especially for treatment by alternative practitioners.

The demand for **supplementary health insurance** in Germany seems to be enormous, as almost every major insurance company nowadays offers such additional plans. Due to the huge selection, it is not easy to find a suitable rate. Therefore, I would like to bring some light into the darkness of alternative practitioner rates in the following.

In Germany, anyone can take out such supplementary insurance, regardless of which health insurance company they are insured with. Furthermore, it should be noted that most insurance companies have a waiting period. Often this is three months. In really good tariffs, not only the alternative practitioner treatments are included, but also glasses and contact lenses, osteopathy treatments and preventive examinations.

A few years ago, when alternative practitioner insurance had just started to conquer the market, many health questions still had to be answered. Currently, most insurance companies limit themselves to about three to four basic health questions.

If you do not have a current or past serious or chronic illness (epilepsy, cancer, multiple sclerosis, etc.), then signing a contract is usually not a problem. Histamine intolerance or irritable bowel syndrome are not among such serious illnesses.

The monthly costs for alternative practitioner insurance can be very different. In addition, the cost of insurance also depends on your age. But if you really want to get your histamine problems under control, you have to rely on a therapist, on lab tests and on medications. Of course, all of this leads to costs that can be covered by such an insurance plan.

Normally, I'm not a big fan of insurances. With most insurance, it is questionable whether you need it at all. Alternative practitioner insurance, on the other hand, is one of the few insurance plans that I think makes a lot of sense. The good thing is that you don't have to pay for the insurance for the rest of your life, but you can cancel it when it is no longer needed. In addition to supplementary insurance, there is another way for reimbursing costs: Via your **tax return**. Healthcare costs cannot be deducted from your tax in every country, but you should definitely check if this option exists.

For the entire histamine intolerance treatment, there are several ways to keep costs within a reasonable range:

- √ Check with your own health insurance company if they cover the required services
- √ If not, try to find appropriate supplementary insurance (if available and cost-effective)
- √ Taxes: It makes sense to check, if services rendered are possibly tax-deductible
- √ If nothing has helped: Ask your health insurance provider for a reimbursement afterwards and an individual case decision

Closing words

We have seen so far: Histamine intolerance is not a very simple topic and there are a few stumbling blocks standing in the way of curing it. But at the same time, there is an enormous number of possibilities nowadays to do something about it. Those who suffered from histamine intolerance 30 or 40 years ago had a much harder time.

And with this guidebook, I hope to contribute to more and more people being well acquainted with the topic of histamine intolerance. Unfortunately, there are too many companies out there that have no interest at all in curing the cause, because no money can be made from healthy people. If there is to be major progress on the subject of histamine intolerance in the future, then it must come from those who are affected. The wider the network of knowledge, the more people with histamine intolerance can achieve together.

The decisive factor for dealing with histamine intolerance is that the body is first able to rest. Therefore, the major factor is to adapt your diet accordingly. This won't certainly be perfect in the beginning and there is no 100% way to avoid histamine. But with an adapted, low-histamine diet, you can already help your body enormously, since it is no longer constantly burdened with a huge histamine surplus.

After the diet has been adjusted and the body has thus calmed down, the next step is to look for the actual root cause. To do this, we have looked at a variety of possibilities, such as checking the DAO value or for missing nutrients, impaired intestinal flora, heavy metals, hormones or even a prolonged intake of a medication.

If it was possible to choose a food intolerance, then a lactose or fructose intolerance would certainly be the better choice. The range of foods you can't tolerate with them is much smaller and easier to understand than with histamine intolerance. Unfortunately, you are not asked which intolerance you would like to have. And besides all the negative things that histamine intolerance brings with it, you can also grow by taking on this task.

Nevertheless, I hope that you will manage the initial change in diet and lifestyle well and that you will not lose heart when there are setbacks. With a little perseverance, you will be able to feast heartily again one day without having to worry about histamine at all.

IBS AND DIGESTIVE DISORDERS
FROM A TOTALLY NEW PERSPECTIVE

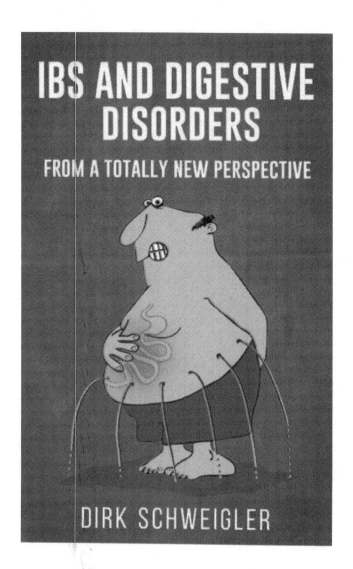

About the author

Dirk Schweigler discovered his passion for writing while he was studying. His diploma thesis was nominated for the *"Friedrich List Prize"* and he has had the opportunity to present his research results at international conferences in Rio de Janeiro as well as in the Netherlands.

Already during his studies, Dirk was fascinated by travel and he backpacked his way several times through Japan, Mexico and the United States. After completing his studies, he wanted to get a new perspective on the world and lived in India for over a year to study the Hindu scriptures. Meanwhile, he has been working as a scientist at a German university hospital for several years now.

Dirk himself was an IBS and histamine intolerance patient for a long time. Since no doctor could help him anymore, he simply took the healing of his intestinal problems into his own hands. For over three years, he tried out many things, carried out intensive research and exchanged ideas with other patients who were also suffering from digestive disorders. Taking this with him to become an author who distinguishes between the symptoms of a disease and the underlying cause, Dirk is excited to share his findings and prove that "just live with it" is never the answer.

Contact:
Dirk.Schweigler@gmail.com

Appendix 1 – Anesthetics, narcotics and X-ray contrast media

Table 4: Charité Berlin University Hospital guidelines for anesthetics, narcotics and X-ray contrast media for patients with mastocytosis and histamine intolerance [22].

Group	Low histamine risk	Higher histamine risk
Benzodiazepine	Diazepam, Midazolam, Flunitrazepam etc.	
Analgesics	Alfentanil, Fentanyl, Sufentanil, Remifentanil	Morphin, Codein, Pethidin, Tramadol
	Paracetamol Naloxon (inhibits the release of histamine)	NSAID, Metamizol
Hypnotics	Propofol, Etomidat, Ketamin	Thiopental, Phenobarbital
Muscle relaxants	Cisatracuronium, Pancuronium, Vecuronium	Atracuronium, Mivacuronium, Suxamethonium, Succinylcholin, Rocuronium
Local anesthetics	Ropivacain, Mepivacain, Bupivacain, Prilocain	Lidocain, Procain, Tetracain
Volatile anesthetics	Enfluran, Isofluran, Sevofluran, Desfluran	
Anticholinergics		Atropin
Plasma Expander		Gelatin, hydroxyethyl starch
X-ray contrast agents		Contrast media containing iodine

Bibliography

1]   Institute of Nutritional Medicine: Nutrition in histamine intolerance. TU Munich. Munich. Available online at https://www.mri.tum.de/sites/default/files/seiten/histamin intoleranz_essen_und_trinken.pdf.

2]   IMD Laboratory: Histamine Intolerance. Berlin. Available online at https://www.imd-berlin.de/spezielle-kompetenzen/nahrungsmittelunvertraeglichkeiten/histami nintoleranz.html.

[3]   Schmidt, R.; Thews, G. (1993): Physiologie des Menschen. 25th ed. Berlin, Heidelberg, s.l.: Springer Berlin Heidelberg.

[4]   Federal Ministry of Health (June 21, 2018): Financial reserves of health insurance funds continue to grow to almost 20 billion euros. Berlin. Available online at https://www.bundesgesundheitsministerium.de/presse/pre ssemitteilungen/2018/2-quartal/finanzreserven-krankenkassen.html.

[5]   Bavarian State Ministry for the Environment and Consumer Protection (2017): Histamine intolerance. Munich. Available online at https://www.vis.bayern.de/ernaehrung/ernaehrung/ernae hrung_krankheit/histamin.htm#diagnostik.

[6]   Swiss Histamine Intolerance Interest Group (SIGHI) (2019): Diagnosis of histamine intolerance. Marthalen. Available online at https://www.histaminintoleranz.ch/de/.

[7]   Beutling, D. M. (1996): Biogenic amines in nutrition. Berlin: Springer.

[8]   Deppe, Kristin (2018): Neue Wege aus dem Histamin-Dilemma. 1st edition. Hamburg: tredition GmbH.

[9]   Biovis Diagnostik MVZ GmbH (2013): Diamine oxidase concentration as a marker of histamine intolerance. Limburg. Available online at http://www.biovis-diagnostik.eu/wp-content/uploads/biovis-DAO-Einzelblatt.pdf.

[10]   IMD Laboratory: Mineral Analysis in Whole Blood. Berlin. Available online at https://www.imd-berlin.de/fachinformationen/diagnostikinformationen/mine ralstoffanalyse-edta-vollblut.html.

[11]   Centrosan: trace element copper. Heerlen. Available online at https://www.centrosan.com/Wissen/Naehrstoff-Lexikon/Spurenelemente/Kupfer.php.

[12]   Fromme, S.: Zink: Das Multitalent. UGB- Verband unabhängiger Gesundheitsberatung e.V. Wettenberg. Available online at https://www.ugb.de/ernaehrungsplan-praevention/zink-multitalent/.

[13]   Deutsche Gesellschaft für Ernährung e.V.: Referenzwerte für die Nährstoffzufuhr. Bonn. Available online at https://www.dge.de/wissenschaft/referenzwerte/.

[14]   Mutter, J.; Haley, B.; Runte, H. R. (2009): Healthy instead of chronically ill! The holistic way: prevention and healing are possible. Weil der Stadt: Fit-fürs-Leben-Verl.

[15]   Lademannbogen laboratory: Diamine oxidase. Hamburg. Available online at https://www.labor-lademannbogen.de/analysen/analysen-spektrum/analysenverzeichnis/analysis/show/alphabetisch es-analysenverzeichnis/diaminooxidase/.

[16]   Weber, M. (2016): Insulin- und seine vielen
Gegenspieler. Ed. by Verlag Kirchheim. Mainz. Available
online at https://www.diabetes-online.de/a/insulin-und-
seine-vielen-gegenspieler-1766724.

[17]   Walter, M., Maaß, H.: Hormones and Histamine
Intolerance. Mettlach. Available online at
https://www.histaminikus.de/histaminintoleranz/192-
hormone-und-histaminintoleranz.html.

[18]   Biovis Diagnostik MVZ GmbH (2013): Hormones in
saliva. Limburg. Available online at http://www.biovis-
diagnostik.eu/wp-
content/uploads/Biovis_Speichelhormone-DE.pdf.

[19]   Spiesz, K. (2011): Histamine intolerance. Ed. v.
Journal of Nutritional Medicine (4). Available online at
https://www.kup.at/kup/pdf/10396.pdf.

[20]   Radiologie.de: Contrast agents in computed
tomography. Heidelberg. Available online at
https://www.radiologie.de/untersuchungsmethoden-im-
uberblick/computertomographie-ct/kontrastmittel-der-
computertomographie/.

[21]   Jarisch, R.; Hemmer, W. (eds.) (1999): Histamine
Intolerance. Stuttgart: Thieme.

[22]   Interdisciplinary Mastocytosis Center Charite: Notes
on anesthesia and surgery for patients with mastocytosis.
Berlin. Available online at http://www.mastozytose-
charite.de/fileadmin/pdf/Hinweise_zu_Narkosen_Operatio
nen_IMCC_v3.pdf.

Made in United States
Orlando, FL
23 March 2025

59738613R00097